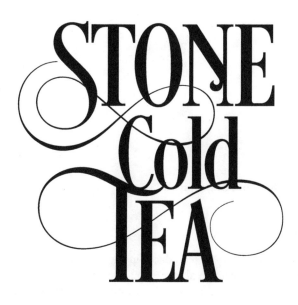

STONE Cold TEA

WINN BRAY RATHBUN

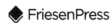 FriesenPress

One Printers Way
Altona, MB R0G 0B0
Canada

www.friesenpress.com

Cover photo: Heather Rathbun-Bishop
Author photo: Thies Bogner

ISBN
978-1-03-919017-7 (Hardcover)
978-1-03-919016-0 (Paperback)
978-1-03-919018-4 (eBook)

1. Biography & Autobiography, Personal Memoirs
2. Health & Fitness, Diseases, Alzheimer's & Dementia

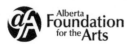 Alberta Foundation for the Arts

Distributed to the trade by The Ingram Book Company

For Mom

To Jenna,

Thank you for coming to my Launch!

CONTENTS

PART ONE

ABANDON

The little blue mug had always been cracked, for as long as I could remember. The chip on the rim still held traces of the last bit of cocoa it had served. I ran my thumb across the picture of the little bear and remembered. Little Punkinhead. Why was he crying?

"Why is he crying, Mommy?"

"He's sad because the other bears won't play with him."

"Why not?"

"Because his hair is so funny."

"It is?"

"Yes. See? It stands straight up and won't lie down."

"Oh." They won't play with him because he looks funny. He's crying.

"Don't send me anything," I told Jayne on the phone. "I don't need anything. Just my Punkinhead mug if it's still there. If it hasn't already been thrown out."

But why this?

I cradled the mug in both hands trying to feel beyond the cool blue paint. What was it about this cheap bit of china? The dirty chip, the long-suffering crack in its side, the cool, smooth blue, and the memory of something warm and sweet inside. Like the wobbling wooden stairs that creaked and weaved as you gingerly made your way to the second-floor cold-water flat. If you can see past the loose steps and the broken front door where the winter wind whistled, don't look at the damp, stained wallpaper. Who could anyway since there is no light in this room? Close the kitchen door where the dishes live on the counter, in the sink, hidden in the gas oven except for those cold days when you sit, all three of you, with your feet up on the open oven door. It was warm. Sometimes, in some of the rooms, if you could see past it all, it was warm. Close off the parts you can't afford to heat. Closed, cool, blue.

"Oh, sure. I remember sitting around that stove," Jayne had said one day when I was trying to evoke positive memories in my sister.

"Sure. It was warm. You said, 'We love you, Mom.' And she smiled. Then I said, 'Well, I adore you, Mom,' and she slapped my face. 'You only adore the Lord!' was her reason. So, I went to bed."

To the cold, closed room. Nothing had been the same for Jayne after that.

*   *   *

Cathy tried to steady the Bible on her lap as the bus jostled along the tree-lined country road. But the words blurred before her and she read more from memory than from sight, each passage comforting her like the feather-down quilt on her bed back home. Bathurst. So far from today.

Dad had been supportive of Cathy's wishes to attend Bible school even if he hadn't quite held with her Evangelical beliefs. "Well Cathy, girl, I know where you get it from. If your mother were alive, she'd approve. You two were quite the Holy Rollers. Ach. The Lord is the Lord, after all. Even if you don't believe he's a Presbyterian."

Oh yes, Mother would have approved. After all, Cathy was working harder in Toronto than she ever had in all her life. Classes, assignments, and housekeeping to pay the tuition, room, and board. Mother would approve, all right.

Another year and a half and she'd be ready for the mission field. China! That would be her mission, God willing. And Sister Pennobecker endorsed.

The bus slowed and chugged uphill, the driver pumping the clutch and pushing it into low gear with a long, painful grind. This little vacation seemed such a waste of time. And there wasn't time to waste. She was already twenty-six. The world was approaching the middle of the twentieth century. Europe was in the throes of war, and scientists had begun to challenge the creation of the world. Everything pointed to the End. Surely the Rapture would soon come. The urgency of it at times made Cathy panic. What if the Lord comes back before I reach my mission? What if I never see China?

"Stop second guessing God," Sister Pennobecker had said. "He'll come in his own time, but you'll be no good to him if you drop dead of exhaustion first. My friends are expecting you. So just go and rest. Refresh."

Cathy closed her Bible with that familiar and comforting thud. Then she prayed, her lips moving just enough to let her words be reflected in the cool window of the chugging bus.

"Heavenly Father, please let there be someone there to meet me in this one-horse town you've sent me to. Help me to see the reason for this trip. Thank you, Lord, for bringing me safely thus far. Thy will be done. And please help this bus make it up the next hill. Amen."

*   *   *

Italian, Hungarian, Ukrainian, and French. Apparently, those were the languages I fit into one sentence the day my parents decided I had better start school soon. State Street in Welland was a veritable League of Nations and as a four-year-old who enjoyed the freedom of playing up and down the street all summer, I was a language sponge. Or so the story goes.

I came home one summer day after playing with the Tullemello kids across the street and the Tomasso girls up the street and could not make myself understood by my parents. I doubt that my friends and I ever spoke anything but English to each other. But I heard them talk with their parents in the language of their homelands, and we were always welcome in the home of Mrs. Pittmann, the German lady next door who kept candy on hand just for us. I don't remember what it was I said that day. I only knew that I understood myself. So did most of my friends.

On the September morning that summer vacation ended and school began, Jayne was to go into grade one, and I would start kindergarten at Central School, which Paul and Jim were already attending. Our brothers would be responsible for making sure their sisters got to school on time each morning. But on the first day, Mom would have to take us to register me for kindergarten. We were out the door and on our way.

Mrs. Tomasso, two doors down, was also getting her girls off to school. But why, she wanted to know, was I going?

"She's only four, isn't she?"

Mom was always skittish and a little perturbed when people asked such personal questions. She had a habit of assuming that others didn't possess the good manners to mind their own business.

"Yes. But she'll be five in March."

"She can't go to school yet."

"She most certainly can."

"No, Mrs. Bray. She has to be five by February. She'll have to wait another year."

"Another year! Are you sure?"

"Sure, I'm sure. I checked because she's the same age as my Allie. But Allie will be five in December."

"Oh, no." Mom had not expected to have anyone at home with her anymore. She had plans. She was going to work. How was she going to work if I wasn't in school with Jayne?

Mom, Jayne, and I walked to Central School together. Our brothers had gone on ahead. The large brick building stood as it had for decades in the centre of town next to the market between Young and Division Streets. Years later Mom would tell me that our dad had attended this same school when he was a boy and at a time when schools in Welland were few and far between. He must have gone in that same door where all the boys were lined up now. We couldn't see Paul or Jim. Or maybe they didn't want us to see them. We walked over to the other side of the school where all the girls were lined up, and Jayne hugged me goodbye.

"Be a good girl, now, and listen to your teacher," Mom advised.

"I will!" She seemed so ready for whatever excitement grade one had to offer. A bell rang and the two lines of trusting children disappeared into two opposite sides of the school.

"Well, come on, then." Mom took me by the hand.

"Where are we going?"

"To get a cup of tea."

We were going to "sit down!" Maybe at Woolworth's lunch counter on Main Street. Or maybe at that restaurant where Dad sometimes bought Jayne and I ginger beer floats! "Sitting down" was always a treat. We walked past the restaurant and on down to Main Street. The Woolworth's lunch counter it is.

Woolworth's floors don't creak. Peoples, further down Main Street, has dull floors made of skinny, wooden boards that creak and squeak when you walk on them. But Woolworth's floors are tile. They don't creak. We pass the cash registers at the front and head over to the long wall where the lunch counter is. Bright lights bounce off all the stainless steel and the whole area smells like food. Egg salad, soup, cupcakes, and Dad's coffee. Mom orders tea for herself.

"And what would you like, Sweetie?" asks the smiling waitress through her lipstick. Her soft, brown hair is short and curly under her little white hat. She looks like a nurse, almost. Her uniform is white except for the collar and trim on the short sleeves, which are the same pale green as the milkshake machine. And she has an apron—a stiff white apron with a ruffle and a bow in back where it's tied.

What would I like? I eye the chocolate cake sitting on a silver pedestal under a glass dome. On the wall, behind the waitress, are cut-out pictures of strawberry ice cream cones and pieces of pie bursting with apples or cherries. What would I like? Further down the counter is the fascinating pop machine—a giant glass ball filled with orange pop that swishes round and round like Dad's lawn sprinkler, tempting you, making you thirsty. I look up at Mom.

"You may have an orange pop, if you like."

"Yes, please! Orange pop, please!"

The waitress smiles at me. "Okay, Sweetie. One orange pop coming right up."

Perfectly pleased with the choice I've made, I swivel in my chair, pushing myself off the counter and surveying the store as I turn. Mom is sitting with her chin on her hand. Elbows on the table! How come she's allowed? Push again and I face the jewelry counter where crystal clip-on earrings and coloured beaded necklaces sit inside square glass bins. Next on my tour is the back of the store which is less interesting. Mostly brooms and kitchen things. All the way back to the lunch counter where my orange pop has magically appeared!

"Oh do stop that spinning, Poodie." Mom pours milk from the small white pitcher into her teacup. Then the tea. She sighs.

"Are you all right, Mrs. Bray?" Our waitress knows Mom.

"Oh yes, Dear. Thank you."

I know she is. She just sighs a lot.

My orange pop fizzles in the glass. Bobbing in the middle is a red and white striped straw. How I love sitting down! I finish my orange pop long before Mom finishes her tea. She has taken a short pencil and a small notebook out of her purse and is writing something. Numbers, maybe. Or the squiggly markings she calls shorthand.

"Would you like more hot water, Mrs. Bray?" The waitress is picking up the small, metal teapot.

"Yes, thank you. My tea has gone cold. Poodie, please stop that spinning!"

I jump down and venture over to the jewelry counter. I can just see into the sides of the glass boxes that sparkle with rainbow-coloured crystals. Further down the aisle sit several black velvet necks with no heads on which are draped double and triple strings of glass bead necklaces. Some are gold and frosted white pearls. There are pale blue and green crystals, with matching earrings and brooches shaped like leaves, butterflies, and sunbursts. They're beautiful. Someday I'll have earrings like that, I think.

"Poodie, *Viens ici!*" Mom likes to speak French in public even though we don't speak French at home. But I know what she means by viens ici. Time to go.

We walk down Main Street toward the lift bridge where we turn and head to our next stop, the library. It's a low brick building right across the street from Merritt Park, facing the canal. Along the side of the building is the outdoor entrance to the children's section where I will pick up two or three small books about Peter Rabbit and sit at the table which is just the right size for me. Mom is upstairs choosing thick hard-cover books that are wrapped in clear plastic and crinkle when you open them. When I finish looking at the pictures and figuring out the stories about Peter, I leave the books on the table and take the inside stairs to the grown-up library. Mom is somewhere between the shelves. She checks out her books, and we head across the street to Merritt Park where she will sit and read in the warm September sun. I dip my hands in the big white fountain, splashing beads of water into the sky. They sparkle in the sun. They look like the crystal necklaces at Woolworth's.

We're home again by the time Jayne gets back from school with Jim and Paul. She's excited about having made a new friend who lives right across from the school and about sitting in a real desk with a top that opens like a lid. She says that's where they keep their pencils, scribbler, and brand-new spelling book. They're going to start spelling by the end of the week!

"Go on upstairs with you, now. I have to start supper for your father."

Dad will be home soon. Paul and Jim have already disappeared to somewhere. The back yard, maybe.

By the time Friday comes, we have settled into a kind of routine. Once my brothers and sister have left for school, Mom clears away the cereal bowls, sits down with a pot of tea, and I settle on the living room rug to colour for a while. Eventually it's time for both of us to leave the house and head around the corner to the second-floor union hall where Mom has a part-time job cleaning. She empties ashtrays, wipes down desks and long tables, sets chairs straight, and deposits empty pop bottles in the wire rack attached to the bright red Coca Cola machine. If you had a nickel, you could buy a cold bottle of Coke. You dropped the coin in the slot on the front of the machine and pushed a magic button. The bright red machine would chug and then, plop! A small glass bottle of pop would drop into the opening at the bottom. It was cold and sometimes wet. There was a bottle opener on the front of the machine and when you got the cap off the Coke, a small puff of cold steam would fizz out of the bottle. Coca Cola never tasted as good as it did out of those small glass bottles—if you had a nickel.

Sometimes, depending on the day, we'd head over to the library if Mom had finished all her books and needed more. Or sometimes we'd just head back home to our house around the corner where Tinker Toys and Freshie waited for me. I don't know what waited for Mom.

Our house was half a duplex with a deep front porch that we shared with the Leon's office next door. Leon's had their furniture store on the corner of State and King Streets, and they owned our house too. The ladies who worked in the office next door were always very friendly to me. Even when I was asked to please stop jumping up and down on the shared front porch, I was asked in a kind and friendly way.

On warm days, I played outside with the other kids who weren't yet old enough for school. Up and down State Street we'd ride our tricycles. Or maybe we'd jump rope or make mud pies in our back yard. Our back yard had a swing set, but it also seemed to have a fair bit of mud. Alongside the house the delivery trucks for Leon's would pull up to load and unload. It was also where the shiny canteen truck would park. That was always fun to watch. The driver of the canteen truck would open its side panels and pour hot coffee or cold pop out of fascinating spigots that were built right into the truck. Sometimes the salesmen from Leon's would also buy sandwiches for their lunch. Or they might just stand next to the truck, talking to the canteen man and having a smoke.

The side of Leon's furniture store faced State Street and there was a door where sometimes a man, who looked very much like Dad, would stand and smoke. I didn't know his name, but I thought of him as Mr. Leon. If I happened to be riding by on my tricycle when he was there, he would sometimes stop me and give me a quarter to spend around the corner at Betty's or at Bitando's candy store. I really liked Mr. Leon. He always had a smile for me.

Fall became winter became spring. The school routine continued but some things changed. Jayne didn't talk about her pencils, scribbler, or brand-new spelling book anymore. And her new friend who lived across from the school had died in a fire the day after Jayne attended her birthday party. She didn't talk about that much, either.

On a hot and sunny June day, Jayne stood in front of Mom and Dad, who were sitting at the kitchen table. I was told to wait in the living room while they opened my sister's Progress Report from Grade One, but I could still hear what they were saying. Mom was reading the report out loud.

"Miss Black says that your printing needs improvement. That's the same report she gave you in December. I've gone over and over this with you. We even bought you your own blackboard to practice on. Haven't you been practising?"

"Yes." Jayne's voice is unusually meek. "It's just hard to make the letters the way she wants them."

"She wants them the correct way."

"I tried. I just can't. It's too hard with my right hand. And when I do it with my left, she says I'm wrong."

Mom continued. "She also says that your spelling has not improved at all and that you don't take an interest in reading. I can't believe that a child of mine doesn't like to read."

"I *do* like to read," Jayne protests. "I just don't do it as fast as everybody else."

"Well, you need to try a little harder if you want to keep up. She's given you a 'Satisfactory' for behaviour. I should hope so! But an 'Unsatisfactory' for effort and preparedness."

I could see my sister just inside the kitchen doorway slump against the wall, her head down in what looked to be defeat.

Mom continued, "Well, here's the result."

Now I heard our dad. "What does it say, Cathy?"

"This pupil is to . . . be retained in Grade One."

I heard my dad sigh. "I'm sorry Jaynie."

Jayne lifted her head. "What does that mean—retained?"

Mom answered, "It means you have to repeat grade one."

"What?! No! I don't want to. I hate that class. I hate Miss Black! She's mean and she's crazy!"

"Stop that right now," Mom said at the top of her speaking voice.

"She is! She is! She told us that white bread was good for us, but toast was like poison. She did! One day she got mad because somebody fell asleep at their desk, and she made all of us stand up and then she turned all our desks upside down. All of them! We had to stand up until recess!"

Then Dad said, "Jaynie, you mustn't talk about your teacher that way."

"Even if it's true?"

Mom interjected, "Your teacher's behaviour is not the point. Your failure to keep up is. You'll have to try harder next year. You don't want people to think that you're lazy or stupid, do you?

Now Jayne's voice took on a more familiar combative tone.

"I'm not stupid! I'll just look stupid. Daddy, please. Don't let them make me repeat. It's embarrassing. All my friends will be going into Grade Two without me!"

"Surely not *all* your friends." Mom said.

"No, not all." Jayne turned on Mom. "One of them is dead!"

Now Dad spoke up again. "You will not speak to your mother in that way."

"But Daddy!"

"You will not," he repeated.

Jayne let out a frustrated growl that bordered on desperation and cried out, "Oh, Daddy!" She ran out of the kitchen, around the corner, and up the stairs to our bedroom. I heard her slam the door.

Then Mom said, "That little brat!" and made a move to follow. But Dad took her by the arm and said, "Don't, Cathy. Just let her be."

"But Herb—"

"Let her steam," he said. "She's scared and upset. Just let her be."

They turned back into the kitchen where Dad filled his coffee percolator. Mom put the kettle on for tea.

The storm seemed to have passed so I went upstairs and opened our bedroom door. Jayne was pulling things out of our dresser and throwing them on the bed. Shorts, socks, a tee-shirt, her pyjamas.

"What are you doing, Jaynie?" I asked her.

"Leaving!"

13

"Where are you going?"

"To Aunt Minnie and Uncle Peter's."

"To the farm?"

I loved the farm. The long, shady lane that led to their little white house. The huge, airy barn that always smelled of hay. I loved how the cows roamed from the back of the house to the distant tree line and how the chickens just went where they pleased. In spring, there were daffodils and little white flowers everywhere. It was a great place to run free. And if you got too hot you didn't even have to go into the house for a drink. You just pumped the pump and cold, cold water poured out. As much as you could want or need.

"I want to go too!" I said.

Jayne had taken the lid off our Tinker Toy tube and was dumping out all the sticks and wheels.

"Okay!" she said, defiantly. "Grab your pyjamas."

She started shoving her clothes into the empty Tinker Toy tube.

"Can I bring my Koala?"

"She won't fit in the tube. You'll have to carry her," Jayne said.

"Okay." I answered, trying to sound just as determined as my sister.

I had always had my Koala. She didn't have a name, but I knew she was a she because she had a little baby Koala that she carried on her back. It was held there by a big elastic band so that I didn't lose it. Daddy said that Koalas carried their babies in the front, not behind. But that made it hard to cuddle her close. And I never went to sleep without cuddling my Koala. So I would carry her myself.

Jayne shoved my pyjamas into the tube and squished everything down with the tin lid.

"Come on," she said.

"Okay!"

When we got to the bottom of the stairs, Mom and Dad were standing in the kitchen doorway. Dad was holding a mug of coffee.

"What are you two doing?" Mom demanded.

"We're leaving!" Jayne snapped back.

"And just where do you think you're going?" Mom demanded.

"To Aunt Minnie and Uncle Peter's where there's no school and no progress reports and no stupid blackboards!"

"Are you leaving too Pooh?" Dad wanted to know.

"Yes. Pooh too."

"Aren't you coming too, Daddy?" I asked.

"No, not today."

"Of course not," Jayne said to me. "We're running away."

"We are?" That thought had not occurred to me.

"Yes." She grabbed my hand and led me through the kitchen and out the back door. "Come on. Let's get our tricycle."

"Okay." I answered, somewhat less definitively.

Jayne pulled our tricycle out from behind the porch stairs and pushed it across the grass to Leon's back driveway.

"You stand on the back, Pooh, and keep the tube from falling over."

I stepped up onto the back foot-panel and pushed the tube that held all our worldly possessions forward so that it was squished between me and the seat of the tricycle. With one arm I held onto my sister. With the other I held on to Koala and her baby.

"Let's go!" Jayne said, and she pedalled us all the way down Leon's driveway to the State Street sidewalk. There she stopped, turned her head and yelled, "Goodbye forever!"

Goodbye forever? Did she say forever? Suddenly I felt a rush of fear.

"Aren't we going home anymore?" I asked the back of her head.

"No." she grunted. Pedalling down the driveway had been a lot easier than pedalling along the sidewalk with me standing on the back of the tricycle.

I looked back at the house to see if Mom and Daddy were watching us. They were not. Jayne was still grunting and pushing the pedals. We were halfway along the side of the Leon's building slowly making our way to King Street.

"Do you know how to get there?" I asked my sister.

"We turn this corner. Then we go up that street."

"All the way to the bridge? Do we have to cross the bridge?"

"Yes." She gasped, almost out of breath.

"What if there's a boat and the bridge goes up?"

"We wait."

"Then what?"

Jayne stopped pedalling. "It's too heavy. You have to get off."

"Why?"

"It's too heavy! You have to walk."

"All the way?"

"You don't have to come. Go back if you want to, but I'm leaving."

"How far is it?"

Suddenly, it seemed as if all the steam had gone out of her anger. Hands still on the tricycle, Jayne dropped her head and sighed.

"Jaynie?" I asked again. "How far is it?"

"Too far," she replied. Then she got off the tricycle, turned it around and looked at me. "Come on, we gotta go back."

"Okay," I answered, somewhat relieved. "But we'll go another time, right? We'll go to Aunt Minnie and Uncle Peter's farm?"

"Sure," my sister answered. "Someday."

"Okay!"

*   *   *

"Just keep walking. I'm right behind you."

Jayne and I are hand in hand leading the way to who knows where. Mom is taking us for a walk while Dad is at work. It's summer now so who knows where our brothers might be. But Jayne and I are taking a walk with Mom, going somewhere `special.'

We've never gone this way on Main Street before. We always head toward the canal, the lift bridge, and the park. There's a store we've never seen before. This is all new to us.

Something smells wonderful. "Look Mommy, a restaurant." Maybe we're going to sit down.

"Yes, it's a fish and chip shop."

"Is that all they have?" Jayne wants to know.

"Yes, fish and chips. Like at home."

"Home?"

"My home." Ah. She means Scotland.

"All right now. We're going this way."

It's a long road that rolls up and down and winds its way along the river. The tall trees that grow on one side of the road in peoples' front yards speckle the summer sunlight on the sidewalk and provide intermittent cooling shade for our journey. Our seemingly endless journey.

Jayne is more curious than I am. Either that or she's becoming impatient.

"Where are we going?"

"To see a house," Mom answers.

"Why?"

"Because we might live there." Mom is looking straight ahead but Jayne and I look at each other.

Live there? What did she mean, live there? Why would we do that? Jayne has no compunction in demanding information.

"Why would we live there? What's wrong with our house?"

"I said we *might* live there. There's nothing wrong with our house, but it's not ours. This one would be our own home."

We keep a steady pace ahead of our mother but now we have to stop from time to time to comment and evaluate the possible houses. Brick houses. Tall houses. Double houses like ours.

"Look at that one. It's a mansion." Jayne agrees with me. I think it looks scary, but she thinks it is beautiful.

We walk up another hill and cross a driveway that curves round to a low brick building. "That would be your school if we move."

It doesn't look anything like Central School. I thought I was going to go to Central School. We cross the other end of the curved driveway.

"Here we are."

It's big. A big white house with a roof shaped like a barn. There's a wide porch, a giant front lawn, and trees! Giant Christmas trees all along the front of the yard. There's a side yard too. The house that might be our home sits on the corner. A long straight street on one side and our future school on the other.

Jayne is immediately in love. "Mommy, it's perfect!"

"Do you like it?"

"Oh yes. Yes."

What about you, Poodie? Do you like it?"

I don't know if I like it or not. But Jayne does.

"I like it," I say. "I can tell my friends that you have to cross two streets to get to our new house."

"No! You mustn't tell anyone. You mustn't say anything about this house. Not to anyone. Do you understand?"

We're a little puzzled by our mother's sudden anger. Or is it fear? Hard to tell. But we know she is deadly serious.

"Yes, Mommy."

"Not a word. And when we go inside, you are not to say anything. You are to be seen and not heard. Do you understand?"

We've heard that before and we understand.

"Yes, Mommy."

We walk up the front steps as the door opens. A woman greets us.

"Mrs. Bray. Please come in."

She leads us from space to large, airy space, each one empty of furniture. A front room, a dining room in the middle of the house with a large bay window, and another room off the dining room.

"This could be a bedroom, Mrs. Bray." Mom nods approval.

Beyond that is the kitchen with a door that leads to another porch on the side of the house. Then back to the front and up the stairs to the second floor. There's an open landing that would be "perfect as a sewing room." Our mom doesn't sew, as far as we know. There's a bedroom with one window and a ladder built into the wall that leads to the attic. "Lots of storage in the attic." The largest room is on the corner of the house with one big window out front and another window on the side that has a large windowseat.

"This was my son's room, Mrs. Bray, and would be perfect for your girls." Jayne squeezes my hand. This would be our room. And off "our room" is the only bathroom.

"You have to go through this bedroom to get to the bathroom?" Mom inquires.

"Yes. That's why I thought this room would be better for your girls. At their age they need less privacy than the boys."

"Yes, I see what you mean."

Jayne squeezes my hand again and whispers, *our room.*" Mom hasn't heard. Good.

"You girls go out onto the porch now. I need to speak with Mrs. Brook."

"Okay!" And we're gone.

Sitting on the steps of the front porch we begin to plan out the spaces of our soon-to-be new home.

"Do you think we can bring our swing set with us, Jaynie?"

"Of course."

"And our toys?"

"We'd better. And our tricycle."

"Yeah, our tricycle."

We run through an inventory of the important aspects of our lives. Toys, friends, candy stores, and the new distance to Cross Street Pool. Jayne gets up and walks down the steps. She turns to look at the big white house and then the one on the other side of the street. "They're the same," she says, looking back and forth between the two houses.

"What?" I get up and join her on the sidewalk.

"Look. This house and that house are almost the same."

"No."

"Yes. Same roof. Same size."

I look more carefully to try and see what she sees.

"Different porch," I offer.

"Yeah. And it's darker than our house."

She's right. It has more trees and darker paint.

"Yeah."

"I like our house better." Jayne decides.

"Me too." I have to agree with my sister. She's almost always right.

Mom steps out onto the porch, turns, and thanks Mrs. Brook, then comes down the steps to meet us on the walk. She takes each of us by the hand and we head off. She doesn't even turn back to see the big white house once more. But we do. Jayne and I crane our necks to get one last look at what could be our new home.

The trip back to Main Street seems shorter. Maybe because Mom is keeping a pretty brisk pace. And she's humming to herself.

"Well, girls. What did you think?"

"Can we bring our swing set?" That's my main concern.

Mom laughs. "Yes, Poodie. If we move there, you can bring your swing set."

Then Jayne shares our opinion. "Ours is the nicer house, Mommy."

"What do you mean?"

"The house on the other side of the street is almost the same but darker."

"The porch is different, too!" I add, not to be outdone in observation.

"Yes," Mom hesitates then says, "That's where your father's cousins live."

"They do? I didn't know Daddy had cousins.

"Oh, yes. He does."

"Are they our cousins, too?" I ask.

"In a way, Poodie. Second and third cousins."

I don't know what that means but the question disappears from my head because now we are stopping in front of the fish and chip shop.

"Are we going to sit down, Mommy?"

"Yes, let's treat ourselves to dinner."

The green, wooden screen door to Ideal Fish and Chips opens with a welcoming creak and we go in. There are a few tables and chairs and a long counter where a pile of newspapers lays. Beside them stand two large canisters with handles. One for salt. One for pepper. The smell of fried batter, fish, and hot oil overwhelms our senses. Right there, behind the counter, a man in a dirty white apron plunges a wire basket down into hot sizzling oil, then turns to us with a smile.

"Eat in or take out?" he wants to know.

"We'll eat in, thank you, Louie. In the dining room, please."

"Sure. This way." He wipes his hands on his apron and leads us past the counter and the vats of hot oil to the back of his establishment.

There are two adjoining rooms back here. The wooden walls are painted a flat, pale green and from the ceiling bright, bare light bulbs hang from long black cords. Mom moves to the room further from the front and chooses a table with four chairs.

"Thank you. This will be fine."

"What would you like to drink, Ma'am?"

"A pot of tea, please. And cream soda for the girls."

Cream soda? Jayne sees my quizzical look.

"It's red pop," she whispers.

"Oh. Okay!"

On the table are salt and pepper shakers and a bottle of vinegar as well as knives, forks, and paper napkins for each of us. A different person comes back with our drinks. He's younger and has a clean apron. Maybe he doesn't do the cooking.

"Two orders, please," Mom says to him. "One for me and one for the girls to share."

"Yes, Ma'am."

The red pop is cold and welcome after our hot summer hike.

"Don't gulp it, Poodie. Save some for your dinner."

The next thing to arrive is small plate with soft white bread and a dish of real butter. At home, it's my job to knead and mix the yellow colouring through the bag of white margarine to make it look like butter. But this is real butter. And the bread is so soft! Now that the waiter has left, we can talk about the house. Jayne is visibly excited.

"Mommy, it's perfect. I can't wait to live there."

"It's not ours yet. And remember, you are not to say a word to anyone about it."

"Not even Jim and Paul?"

"No, Poodie. No one."

"I'm glad you found that house, Mommy." Jayne is beaming.

"Me too!" I agree with my sister.

"How did you know it was there, Mommy?"

"I've seen it before."

"When?"

"A long time ago."

The pictures formed perfectly in her mind now. She could see the second-floor bedroom where Sister Pennobecker's friend had put her up. The wood-frame bed, the hardwood floor, the teddy bears and dolls that sat expectantly on the cedar chest beneath the dormered window. They had been expecting a younger girl, it seemed. What a shock she must have been to Ernie and Maggie when they met her at the bus, in her fashionable wool suit, matching green hat and shoes.

"Cathy Smith?" Maggie asked tentatively when she was the only one to get off the bus.

"Yes. From Toronto."

"She's not a girl!" blurted young Ernie.

"Quiet!" snapped Maggie. "We gotta walk." Maggie apologized, looking down at the high heels.

"It's about two miles. I'm Maggie. This is my cousin, Ernie. Mom and Grandmother Rose are waiting at the house."

"Thank you. I love to walk."

She handed Ernie her bag and fell into step with the young girl.

"Hey!" Ernie's protest was answered with a frown from Maggie which clearly meant 'Shut up, Ernie.'

If Cathy was a surprise to this family, Grandmother Rose was a shock to Cathy. She hadn't seemed quite real from a distance, so still had she stood on the porch like the main pillar that held up the dark homestead. Grandmother Rose was a figure frozen in time.

She assessed Cathy from a distance, taking note of her tall stature, the hat, Ernie carrying her bag. Were those high heels? And the tailored green suit fit much too closely. It emphasized a slender waist, shapely legs, and a far too prevalent bosom. Could this young woman really be a future missionary? Grandmother Rose had her doubts.

The closer they drew the more formidable the matriarch seemed to Cathy. Grey hair pulled back in a tight, neat bun. Thin lips pulled back too, in a stern and unforgiving line. And pale, calculating eyes assessing the guest. And yet, when she spoke it was with a warm and welcoming voice.

"How do you do, Miss Smith. We're very glad to welcome you to our home."

"Thank you. You're very kind." Perhaps it would be fine after all.

Now Maggie sat cross-legged on the bed watching Cathy's every move. A young girl just beginning to think about being a woman, her eyes roamed lovingly over each item as Cathy unpacked her travelling bag. A small hand mirror, hairbrush, white cotton gloves, and lace hankies. All the accoutrements of womanhood.

"I'm going to have lace hankies someday."

"I'm sure you are."

Cathy took a small white bundle from her case and unwrapped her bottle of Evening in Paris perfume, a gift from Dad last Christmas. She set the small blue bottle on the highly polished dresser and smoothed the deep blue tassel tied around its neck. The bottle was nearly full still. Perfume was meant to be saved for special occasions like Christmas, the theatre, or visits to small, strange towns where there was absolutely nothing to do.

"What's that?" Maggie inched forward on the bed.

"Perfume."

"Can I smell it?"

Cathy picked up the bottle, gently twisted off the top, and placed it under Maggie's nose.

"Oh! That's strong!"

"Well, you're only supposed to use a little. And not every day."

She put the perfume back on the dresser. Perching on the window seat, Cathy bent down and unbuckled each lovely shoe, then stretched out her feet and wiggled her crooked toes.

"You must be tired. I should go and let you rest before dinner."

"No need."

"I have to go down and set the table anyway."

And she was gone.

Cathy picked up her shoes and placed them beside the bed. What a lovely quilt. Soft and thick with feathers. The bed was narrow but firm. Quite comfortable. Quite soothing after that endless journey. Perhaps she would read a bit before dinner. The sun was just beginning to set. Her feet were a little sore after all.

Perhaps she would just close her eyes for a moment.

"Will that be all, Mrs. Bray?"

Mom snaps back out of her daze.

"Yes, thank you."

The tall man in the white apron puts the paper check on our table and leaves. Mom takes a wallet from her purse and begins to count out a couple of dollar bills and a few coins.

"How does he know your name, Mommy?" I ask.

"Everyone knows Mommy," Jayne explains.

But our mother corrects her. "Not me. It's your father he knows. I'm just Herb Bray's wife. But everyone loves Herb Bray."

"They do?"

"Well, he's lived here all his life."

And I think to myself, well, where else would he live?

*   *   *

Our new home was wonderful and so much larger than the house on State Street. On moving day, Jayne and I ran through each room giggling and spinning like the ballerinas we knew we'd grow up to be. From the front room, through the archway to the wide hall and into the middle room with the big bay window. The room off that was our parents' bedroom. We didn't go in there. The kitchen at the back was less interesting but it led out to the side door and porch. Down the steps to the end of the walk where a gigantic mulberry tree nobly stood, sharing and shedding its fruit. Back up the walk and around the house to a huge, green yard. Grass, in such short supply on State Street, rolled out before us and ran the length of the house through an opening in a tall hedge and all across the front yard. More trees! One, two, three, four evergreens from the fence of the school next door right to the other corner of our yard. Here lived another tree, abundant with little red berries, which we soon learned were very sour. But the birds feasted there, heartily. Back up the front stairs and across the wide porch we danced. Back at the front door now, we turned the little metal lever which rang an actual bell on the other side, opened the door and ran up the stairs that were right there to our left. This is Jim and Paul's room. This is Mom's sewing room. And THIS is our room, the biggest and best in the whole house, in our new home.

Furniture began to arrive. Familiar things from the old house like the grey chrome kitchen table and matching padded chairs. The yellow, vinyl stool that you were not supposed to poke holes in with a needle no matter fascinating the sound was. Our parents' bedroom furniture and our brothers' bunk beds. Then there were the unfamiliar things needed to fill the big new house.

The middle room was transformed with the arrival of a matching dining room suite. There was a wooden table that would sometimes be round and sometimes be oval because it had leaves. Not tree leaves like in our yard. Wooden leaves that made the table longer. There were six matching chairs. One chair had arms and would sit at the head of the table. That was our dad's. There was a tall china cabinet with a glass door and a little brass handle. That would hold our mom's better dishes.

And there was a long buffet sideboard with doors and drawers that sat along the far wall of the newly christened dining room. The room where our family was going to dine every day. I don't know where all this furniture came from.

But our favourite piece, Jaynie's and mine, was the new-to-us four-poster bed. A great big, beautiful bed of our very own for our great big, beautiful bedroom. The best room in the house.

The front room had our old couch which sat under the big, flat window and a new La-Z-Boy chair, just for our dad. This special piece of furniture was placed at one end of the room facing our long-legged television at the other.

Mom knew the lady across the street from our new home because they both attended services at the Salvation Army. From her we acquired the piano and bench. It was wonderful too. An old upright Grand of deeply coloured wood that gleamed with years of buffing and care. The front of it was beautifully sculpted and boasted two hand-carved candle holders, one on either side of the sound board. It was placed in our front room flat against the shared wall of our parents' bedroom. When you sat at the piano, sunlight from the big front window warmed your back. Aside from our four-poster bed, this would become my favourite place to sit, next to my dad as he played. Mom said he didn't need to read music like the lady at church because he played by ear. He said maybe I could too. So, he told me to listen to the melody as he played it. Then he showed me what keys to play. One finger, one note. Next finger, next note, until I made a melody too. We played it together. He said I had an ear for music. I knew I had two.

A girl named Betty from up the street came to our door often, especially on weekends, to ask if she could walk our dog, Caesar. More often than not our big brother Jim was, "just about to walk him myself. Want to come along?"

I didn't understand why you would need two people to walk our dog. But Betty and Jim seemed to think you did. So off they would go together with Caesar on a long leash for a longer walk.

Caesar had come into our family from the local Humane Society shortly after we moved into the house on River Road. I don't know whose idea that was, but I do know that Jim really wanted a hunting dog. What he got was a five-year-old black and white Dalmatian that apparently really didn't want to be adopted. Or maybe he just didn't want to live with us, because he kept running away. And not just out into the woods or someone else's yard. Our dog would run back to the Humane Society. He would flee through muddy banks all the way along the edge of the Welland River toward the aqueduct. There he would cross over the river to the island that sat between the river and the Welland Canal. That was where the Humane Society had its shelter.

The first time he was found barking at the shelter door, our dad got a call reminding him that we couldn't just give the dog back. The second time he ran away, Dad knew where to find him. After the third trip to retrieve our dog, Dad decided that Caesar's freedom needed to be limited until he learned to obey.

Dad ran a long clothesline from one of the tall evergreens in the front yard, through the break in the hedge beside the house, all the way to the garage. On a collar and long leash, Caesar had a run of about a hundred feet. That should have solved the problem. It did not. One day when Betty and Jim went into the yard to get Caesar and take him for a walk, all they found was his collar, still buckled and attached to the leash hanging from the line. Our dog, apparently, was an escape artist.

Mom had named him Caesar in an attempt to make him seem regal. And he really was a lovely looking dog. Trim, tall, and beautifully spotted. But after his final escape—which had rivalled Houdini—Dad decided that our dog was determined to be discontent and renamed him Caesar Disgustus.

In time Caesar gave up his attempts to escape. He learned to accept us, our yard, and his new life as the family dog, sitting with Dad in the living room, riding in Paul's rowboat on the river, hunting ducks with Jim, and standing patiently in the large metal wash tub set out in our yard while Jayne and I gave him baths, soaping, rinsing, and soaping him again and again. Jim's dog. Our pet.

Our big yard was always a hub of activity, from the parade of kindergarten kids, whom I invited through to observe our dad's daffodils, to the full-blown race of abandon that encompassed the entire neighbourhood on one particular summer's day.

Kids' names like Robin, Danny, Mary Jane, and Peter come to mind. I'm sure there were other, older kids, too. I'm fairly certain Paul was there with his buddies. And I'm quite sure that Jim was not. I don't know what game we were playing. It seemed to be a neighbourhood crusade of some sort. Some primeval hunt or campaign of exploration. Whatever it was it took in the whole neighbourhood—street, sidewalk, school, and private yards included.

The adventure involved racing down Almond Street from Ryan's house at one end to ours at the other, running up our driveway, around behind our garage and scaling the chain link fence that bordered Riverview School. Then dropping onto the grass of the schoolyard and making a mad dash back up to the edge of Ryan's house where the race would begin again. There must have been some reason for such a game, but if so, I was blithely unaware of its purpose other than it was fun and exciting.

We had room in our yard for such games. I think it must have been one of the larger yards in the neighbourhood because it housed our garage, our swing set, the sandbox our dad made for us (complete with pulley system crank and cover), a metal barrel for incinerating trash, and Dad's fragrant red rose bush that dispelled any odors from said trash.

All these things were put into service when my siblings and I hosted the Almond Street Carnival featuring Caesar the Wonder Dog, Acrobats, a song-and-dance show, cold grape-flavoured Freshie, and a trip into the haunted garage to "See the Eerie Egress. Only One Penny!"

Because we had our beautiful red, white, and blue wooden batons with sparkling silver balls on top, acquired recently on our trip to the CNE, Jaynie and I had decided that we should use them to put on a show for the carnival. A song and dance like the sister act we'd seen on Ed Sullivan last Sunday night.

The day before the carnival we practised all morning, making up the song and putting it together with movements. We had talked about what the song should be about, and we came up with our very first creation. As I recall, the words and the melody arrived together, and we could hardly wait for our turn to perform.

The day of the carnival, Caesar the Wonder Dog missed his performance, having been whisked away by Betty and Jim for a long walk just as Jaynie and I were getting him into costume. Apparently, hunting dogs don't wear dresses and hats.

29

Nevertheless, our yard began to fill with our friends enjoying the free Freshie and our sandbox (complete with pulley system crank and cover). The swing set was out of service, having had the swings removed to make room for the Acrobats. Paul stood next to the garage door. Above it he had hung a large paper sign on which he'd printed in red paint

SEE THE EGRESS FOR ONLY 1 PENNY!

Above the sandbox din, he could be heard calling out "This way to the Egress! Only one penny to see the mysterious Egress! This way!"

As the Freshie supply began to dwindle, it was time to start the show. First act, the Acrobats! On either side of the empty swing set frame, Jaynie and I each took hold of a crosspiece that held the legs together and climbed up to sit atop. Ta-da! Then we rolled backward, each of us performing a "skin the cat." Ta-da! Now we both reached up and took hold of the top cross bar where the swings usually hung. Hand over hand, we inched our way to the middle where we met. Then Jayne dropped to the ground. Ta-da! I remained hanging for the grand finale. Jayne turned to face me and stretched her arms out in my direction. I pulled myself up, hooked my ankles onto the cross bar, let go, and stretched my body downward, hanging from my ankles. Ta-da! Back up now and one more skin the cat. Then I dropped to the grass below, landing on my feet. Now Jayne and I together, Ta-da! And people applauded!

Our mom came out with more Freshie—orange this time—and I walked over to the garage where a line was beginning to form to see the Egress. I didn't know we had an Egress in our garage, but Paul seemed to know all about it.

"You've never heard of the Egress?" he asked our friends as they handed him their pennies. "Oh, you can't miss it," he said, smiling.

My friend from kindergarten, Peter, handed over his penny and got in line. I kind of liked Peter, and now I thought that he was very brave, too. When there were about a dozen kids gathered, Paul moved to the garage door and spoke out in a loud voice.

"Last chance! Last chance to see the Egress! One show only today. Anyone else? No? Very well."

Then he turned to the kids lined up and said very seriously, "This way. Follow me and do exactly as I say." A dozen small heads nodded, seriously.

He opened the side door to the garage, led the group inside, and closed the door again. I waited but not long. From inside the garage, I heard a collective sigh, mixed with groans and then laughter. The garage door opened and out they poured. I watched our friends, neighbours, and classmates walk away from the garage, some of them shaking their heads, others shrugging their shoulders and heading for more Freshie.

Then I saw Peter. He was standing next to my brother, holding a stick and crying, so I went over to them.

"What's wrong?" I asked Paul.

But it was Peter who answered. Sniff, sniff, sob.

"He stole my penny." He sobbed again and whacked the stick on the ground.

"I didn't steal anything. You paid your penny, and I showed you the Egress."

"You lied! You stole my penny!" he sobbed, whacking the stick with every word.

"Wasn't there an Egress?" I asked.

"Sure," Paul answered. "Egress is Latin for "exit." I showed everyone the exit. They laughed."

"You lied!" Peter shouted.

"I didn't lie. Here's your penny, you big baby. And stop swinging that stick at me." Paul grabbed the stick and broke it in half, which sent Peter into a temper tantrum. He grabbed his penny from Paul's hand and ran from the yard.

Then Paul turned to me. "Is that your friend?"

"Yeah. From school."

"I guess you like him, eh?"

"Kinda."

"See what a baby he is? He cried over a joke and a broken stick. What do you want to like him for?"

"I guess I don't."

"Good. Come on. Do you want to do your song now?" Paul asked.

"Okay." And we moved on with the show.

Jaynie went into the house and brought out our batons. Then Paul called out to everyone to come and sit in front of the swing set to see the rest of the show. Behind them I could see our mom, standing against the house, Freshie pitcher in hand, waiting to hear her girls sing.

Side by side, my sister and I began the show.

Each with a sparkling baton in one hand, we swept our arms up to the sky then down to the ground and sang the first line.

"The heavens open wide, and angels come down from above,"

Again, we swept the batons up and down to the ground with the next line.

"The heavens open wide, and angels come down from above,"

Now there was a change in melody and here, we held our batons beside us like walking sticks and strutted around in a full circle to the left.

"Maybe in that heaven there'll be an angel for you,"

And now a full circle to the right.

"Maybe in that heaven there'll be an angel for me too,"

And once more, with baton in one hand we swept our arms up to the sky then down to the ground as we sang:

"The heavens open wide, and angels come down from above!"

Bow and applause! They liked it. Wow. People never applauded when we sang in church.

Let's do it again!

The heavens open wide, and angels come down from above,
The heavens open wide, and angels come down from above,
Maybe in that heaven, there'll be an angel for you,
Maybe in that heaven, there'll be an angel for me too,
The heavens open wide, and angels come down from above!

*   *   *

"More coffee?" Mom is standing by the stove.

"No. Just hot water."

"Try to eat something, Herb. Toast. I'll make a slice."

"I really don't think I can eat."

"I'll make it anyway. At least you have your lunch for later. Maybe you'll be hungry then."

"Maybe."

There's a long silence in the kitchen where my parents sit at sunrise.

"How are you feeling?"

"How the hell do you think I'm feeling?"

"Sorry."

She mustn't provoke him.

"No. I'm sorry. Tired. That's all. Just tired."

"Long day yesterday. Will you be all right at work?"

"Does it matter? I have to go anyway. Pay for this goddamn house of yours."

"Oh, Herb."

"Well, I do, don't I?"

She searches for a way to change the conversation.

"I made you a meat loaf sandwich for your lunch. Dr. White said you should try to eat more red meat – keep your red cells up. And try to rest."

He doesn't reply.

"Here's your toast. You don't have to leave just yet. Have some jam."

"No wax?" he asks, smiling.

"No. No wax." She sits at the table with him. "What an unprepared bride I was."

"I didn't mind."

"No. You never did." They hold hands.

Mom used to tell the story about the first week of their marriage and the first time she made Dad's lunch for work. She used the homemade jam someone had given them as a wedding gift. The next morning he decided to make his own lunch.

"No," she had protested. "I want to do it for you."

"It's all right, Cathy," he had said. "Let me help a little."

He took the jam jar down from the shelf, opened it, and removed the wax that sat on top of the preserve.

"What's that?" she asked.

"That's the wax, Cathy. The jam is underneath."

It seems she had made him wax sandwiches. This delighted his fellow workers who teased the newlywed, mercilessly. Mom always laughed at herself when she told that story.

"What did I know about being a wife? I couldn't even boil water!"

"Cathy, you know we'll have to talk about the house at some point."

"I know."

"There's not enough in the life insurance to pay off the mortgage."

"I know."

"Maybe we should sell beforehand."

"Our home?"

"The house. Sell while I'm here to help with it."

"We have time. Dr. White said maybe ten years."

"Or maybe three."

"But Herb—"

"Well, who's this coming down the stairs?"

"Oh, no. I'll put her back to bed."

My overly long flannelette pyjama legs fly across the dining room floor and into the dimly lit kitchen.

"I smell toast," I say.

"Yes. That's your father's breakfast."

Dad smiles at me. "Why are you up so early, Pooh?"

"Toast and jam with Daddy."

"Come here Sweetie. Sit on Daddy's lap." He lifts me up.

"Herb—" Mom begins to protest.

"She's hungry," he answers her.

"It's sunrise!"

"And she's hungry. Here Baby. Let's share Daddy's toast. Jam?"

"Yes please. Both sides."

"Yes, certainly, both sides."

Mom sighs. "Oh, what a mess she'll be."

"Is it good?" he wants to know.

"Yes, Daddy. Thank you."

"You're welcome, my little Pooh."

I lay my head on his shoulder, and he laughs then begins to cough.

"Herb, why don't you drive in today? I don't need the car."

"No need. I'll take my bicycle."

"But you're so tired."

"Are you tired, Daddy? Go back to bed," I suggest.

Mom answers for him. "Daddy has to go to work."

"Yes," he adds. "Daddy has to go to work. And I'll ride my bike."

"Daddy," I begin quietly, "yesterday when Miss Johnson was reading and we were all sitting on the floor Debbie Penny said I touched her hair, but I didn't. But she told Miss Johnson I did."

"Why did she think you touched her hair?"

"I don't know. I was sitting behind her, and Miss Johnson said to stop but I never did it. Then Debbie Penny said I did it again and I never. But then, after, Miss Johnson made me move and sit somewhere else."

"After what?"

"After Debbie Penny kept saying I touched her hair, and I didn't know why. So, I did touch it to see why I would have, and then Miss Johnson made me move. Everyone stared at me."

"Maybe you should just stay away from Debbie Penny for a while."

"Okay."

"That's enough now." Mom stands. "Get off Daddy's lap and let him go to work."

"Okay. Bye Daddy."

"Bye my little Pooh. Be good. I'll see you tonight."

We hug and kiss. He lifts me off his lap, stands and picks up his lunch pail.

"Have a good day, Herb."

"We'll talk tonight."

And he's gone.

*   *   *

The early morning train left Welland shortly after dawn. I don't remember how we got from our home on River Road to the railway station. Perhaps Dad drove us in the old Pontiac. Or maybe a neighbour gave us a ride. What I do remember was the excitement we always felt whenever we had the chance to take the train to Toronto.

It was a big step up from the wooden box to the metal train stairs and into the train car itself. The rumbling engine would idle loudly as though impatient to get underway, waiting for us to get up, get in and sit down. There were wide cloth seats that faced each other so that one of you always got to travel backwards. Never Mom, though. Mom could not bear to travel backwards.

The jolt that started the journey pushed our excitement from our bellies into our hearts. Big windows on the world passing by, accompanied by the constant click, click, clicking of metal wheels on the tracks below. You could sit, stretch out, or get up and walk around as the train moved. So much better than a bus. And there was a washroom at the end of the train car that you could only use when the train was in motion; a lesson I learned in the most embarrassing way. No matter. Mom, Jayne, and I were going to the Santa Claus Parade and spending the night at the Ford Hotel.

Arriving at Union Station in Toronto was always such a thrill. You stepped down off the train and onto the long cement platform that led to tall wooden doors at one end. Once through those doors you were in another world. An immense space with the tallest ceiling we'd ever seen, Union Station was a majestic hall of marble, wood, and brass. People everywhere were moving in and out through doors and hallways, beside and around giant pillars, and up and down stairways and escalators.

Down the steps we go to the subway. Mom stops to take three tokens from her change purse and gives us each one.

"Now don't lose it. You need it to get on the subway."

Mom has our suitcase in one hand and me in the other. Jayne follows closely behind me. I clutch the token, ready. We follow a line of people up to the turnstile, deposit our tokens in front of the man inside the glass booth and head toward the subway landing. We are headed north to the Ford Hotel!

Whoosh! Here is our train. The experience is always the same. Always exciting. The doors to the train slide open. We hurry in, find a seat, and sit. Doors close and we're off, rushing from the light of the station into the unknown dark tunnel. Small lights flick past as we speed toward the next stop. The train slows, brakes squeal, and into the light we emerge! Stop. People get off. People get on. We sit. Mom knows where we're going. Each stop is the same until we reach our own destination. Then it's, "Stand up, now. Hurry. Hold hands." The doors slide open and we're off the train.

I don't recall checking into the Ford Hotel. It's possible that since it was still early morning, we simply left our suitcase at the front desk and headed out to claim our spot along the parade route. Which we did.

We found prime seats on the curb on Yonge Street just a couple of blocks from Eatons. Jayne and I pulled our winter coats down around our bottoms, tucked our woolen slacks into our boots, and snuggled close together to sit and wait. Mom stood behind us providing a bit of warmth and a windbreak with her long muskrat coat. She was humming. The excitement was palpable as parade-watchers of all ages and sizes jostled, giggled, whistled, and called out to each other in frosty breaths, their words muted in the cold November air. Finally, faintly, we heard the music of a distant marching band echoing against the cement and sandstone buildings lining the parade route. It had begun!

Here came the first brass band, its musicians all in red, followed by a half dozen odd looking clowns with giant heads. Now pretty girls in red and white hooped skirts with red feathers in their hair, leading the first float. More red and white everything with a fellow way up top sitting on a white horse. He was like a knight in shining armor holding a tall spear behind which flowed a long sign made to look like a banner.

EATONS OF CANADA PRESENTS SANTA'S PARADE TO TOYLAND
"THE ENCHANTED WINDS."

Everyone clapped and cheered the Eatons Santa Claus Parade. Now another half dozen clowns upside down walking on their hands. How do they do that? A second float: Peter Pan and the Pirate. Now a big, blue whale and Geppetto in a rowboat escaping its large open mouth. Pinocchio rides up top.

More clowns pulling a shaky Popeye mini-float. Ali Baba. Arabian Knights. Flimsily clad belly dancers.

"Oh dear," Mom sighs with sympathy. "They must be half frozen!"

Jumbo the Elephant magically rolls down the route without any visible means of push or pull. More pretend horses. More clowns. And a long, long float in several sections celebrating the Wild, Wild

West. Mother Goose rides on the back of a giant white and yellow goose and behind her comes Humpty Dumpty, the Pied Piper, a dozen Little Bo Peeps, Little Red Riding Hood, and the Queen of Hearts, all heading to the enchanted Eatons' Toyland.

Now Mom is jumping up and down. Literally, jumping up and down and mutely clapping her gloved hands.

"Listen! Bagpipes! Oh, the bagpipes!"

This is what she's been waiting for. "Scotland the Brave!" She's bouncing and humming and madly applauding as her counterfeit clansmen march past, led by the tall and imposing pipe major. The tassel of his high, black fur hat swings in time to the music and his tartan kilt swishes rhythmically side to side, majestically dancing behind him. More. Let there be more bagpipes, Mom prays. But all too soon for her they have passed, followed most disrespectfully by Bugs Bunny.

"Oh, that was wonderful." She's crying.

The parade continues in much the same way. White Knights, signs for Eatons, another marching band, and more upside-down clowns.

"See. Their hands are really their feet." Jayne explains. "They just look like they're walking upside down."

Now that she's told me how it's done, I see it clearly.

Another brass band. Several cowboys pretending to ride horses that are really just their costumes. You can see their own feet on the ground. And clowns with plastic heads so large all you see are heads and legs.

Then, from behind the blue and white float depicting Holland, complete with working windmill and a dozen little Dutch boys, the sacred sound returns.

"Oh, good! More bagpipes!" Mom is in her glory.

It's not "Scotland the Brave" this time. I don't know what this music is, but it fills the air just the same. Jayne and I bounce our feet on the pavement in time to the music and Mom's own reverie. For her this is the climax of the parade, even though Santa is still two floats away.

The Cobbler and his elves. More clowns. A winter Princess in a candy-cane castle. Another brass band. And the distant sound of, yes, sleigh bells, teasing our anticipation.

When he finally appears, the crowd waves and laughs and breaks into cheers so loudly overwhelming you can barely hear the jolly old man laughing and calling out "Merrry Christmas! Merrry Christmas everyone!" Like a throne, his huge red sleigh towers magically over rooftops and evergreens. His team of eight reindeer move up and down and up and down as though flying. Their golden antlers glisten in the winter sun. Santa waves both white-gloved hands from one side of the street to the other, to include everyone, laughing then singing along as "Jingle Bells" mysteriously blasts from hidden speakers. Santa! The focus of our Christmas desires. He passes us, and we watch the back of the sleigh begin to disappear in the sea of people that follow him.

"Quickly now, girls. Hold hands."

We join the throng following the firetruck, which has signalled the actual end of the parade. Just a couple of blocks to Eatons. And then we'll see Santa up close.

"Can we stop and look at the Christmas windows?"

"Later. After lunch. We'll see Eatons' and Simpsons' Christmas windows after lunch."

Down Yonge Street, in the front door of Eatons and up the elevator. Mom knows this route like the back of her hand. Eatons Santa Claus Parade is a tradition in our family. First, for Mom and Dad in the years before. Then with her boys. Now with her girls. But always with the same plan.

We're standing in line now. Standing hand in hand. Mom has told Jayne to keep me close and she does. Always. I still remember my big sister insisting on my inclusion in all things.

On a hot summer's day Mom would suggest to Jayne, "Shall we go to the pool?"

"Pooh too?" was my sister's concern.

"Yes, Pooh too."

It was always that way with Jayne. Always, in all things.

Miraculously, Santa was already waiting on the second floor, already on his throne waiting to see us. We knew what we were going to ask for and I would let Jayne do the talking.

We join the long line of hopeful children as it shuffles slowly toward the prize. My bare legs begin to itch against my woolen slacks. Even with our corduroy coats unbuttoned it's hot in the store. But the wait will be worth it once we share our secret Christmas wish with Santa. We're nearly there now. An elf is smiling down at us. She's blond and smells pretty, like one of Mom's Avon fragrances. She takes Jayne by the hand.

"Come on, little girl. You're next."

But I am attached to my sister, and we walk up the red carpet to his throne together.

"Well, well, well!' he bellows. What have we here? Twins?"

We've heard that before and Jayne knows exactly how to answer.

"No. We're fifteen months apart."

"Ho, ho! Fifteen months apart! Well, come on then. Up onto Santa's lap. One knee each."

The fragrant elf helps us up. Santa's suit is soft and smooth, and he smells good, too. Not quite like Dad but almost.

"What are your names?"

"I'm Jayne, with a 'y.' This is my sister, Winnifred."

"And how old are you?"

"I'm eight. She's six."

"Seven in March!" I protest.

"Have you been good girls all year?"

Jayne has no hesitation. "Yes."

But I'm remembering what happened with the coins. The day I discovered nickels, dimes, and quarters in a small vase on the windowsill. It never crossed my mind that it belonged to anyone. It was free money. My first taste of personal affluence. So I took it. I kept it. Then I spent it. Or rather, I had a friend spend it for me, because I very quickly learned that if you have money to spend you can pay someone to do things for you. Like go to the store and buy bubble gum for you. So, I'm remembering that when my young enterprise was discovered I was accused of stealing. Apparently, the small vase was Mom's private bank where she saved extra coins for special things, like trips to Toronto to see the Santa Claus Parade. Had I been a good girl all year? How could I answer that?

Jayne answers for me. "We've both been good."

"Well, then. Tell Santa what you would like for Christmas."

"A walking doll," Jayne says.

"A walking doll. That's a lovely gift."

Then he turns to me. "Do you want a walking doll too?"

"Yes, please."

"Well, we'll see what we can do. Two walking dolls for two good little girls."

Wait. That's not right. He hasn't got it right.

"No, not two," I say.

Jayne explains. "Just one for us to share."

We know that two was an extravagance we could never hope for. But Santa isn't listening. The fragrant elf is lifting us off his lap and handing us each a candy cane. The visit is over. Now what? Mom is waiting at the end of the carpet.

"Did you talk to Santa?"

"Yes."

"Good. Let's go have some lunch."

We knew what that meant—the Eatons' cafeteria, where you could pick anything you wanted from a long line of delicious looking sandwiches, salads, and cookies all displayed on shining stainless steel under glass! But best of all, red and green Jell-O cut into amazing square chunks, served in little goblet-like glass dishes and topped with real whipped cream. The walking doll worry was forgotten.

We followed the plan. A cafeteria lunch. Then back out into the winter air to see the Christmas windows. Eatons first, then Simpsons. Amazing, moving displays of magic captured our imaginations like a front row puppet show with no strings. There were beautiful dolls that danced. Small musicians that bowed violins and raised trumpets to their lips. And trains that ran around, under and through papier mâché mountains that were covered in little Christmas trees and sparkling snow.

All along the street and around the corner, every window told a different story of Christmas from the birth of Christ to the emancipation of Rudolf. There, displayed in full living motion were all the wonderful things we could covet, dream of, and purchase at the T. Eaton Company store with a guarantee of joy from Punkinhead, the company's honourary marketing elf.

Only when the afternoon began to fade did our enthusiasm wane. It had been an early morning, an exciting afternoon, and a long day. We arrived back at the Ford Hotel just in time to consider dinner at Murphy's, a real sit-down restaurant attached to the hotel. This was a treat, also part of the annual plan.

But first things first. Hot tea for Mom. I don't remember what we had for dinner. I don't think it mattered much, so happy were we to just be there. As Jayne and I tucked into bed on either side of Mom that night, we floated off to sleep wrapped in Christmas dreams and clean white sheets.

Morning brought a chance to use the shower! It was only big enough for one person at a time which in itself was a wonderful thing. At home we had a cast iron tub and, as children, Jayne and I shared our bath time. But not at the Ford Hotel.

Mom first. Then Jayne. Then me. Oh, it was amazing. The shower itself stood in the corner of the bathroom, a curved wall made of small black and white tiles. White porcelain handles stuck out from the long, copper pipe that rose up and over your head and ended in a flat, copper shower head. There was a curtain made of rubber that hung from a curved bar, clipped there with odd looking metal rings.

Mom turned on and adjusted the taps and I stepped into the luxury of falling water. It was wonderful, like the fountain in the middle of the Cross Street wading pool only gentler and warm. There was a small square bar of soap and a soft white face cloth, and I luxuriated in both like Cleopatra or the Queen of Sheba until Mom reached in and turned off the taps. All too soon my time was up. We dressed then Mom brushed and braided our hair. Time to go.

Next to the Ford Hotel was the Greyhound bus terminal that boasted a lunch counter and served a limited menu for breakfast. Perched up on the round, vinyl stools we ordered toast, tea, juice, and two individual boxes of cereal, the kind that opened on the side so you could pour milk into your own personal cardboard breakfast box. Mom paid with coins—nickels, dimes, and quarters.

Our train didn't leave until later in the afternoon so that meant we had time to explore Yonge Street. Mom checked our suitcase in a locker at the bus station and we headed out to the stores. Most fascinating to me was the wooden escalator in either Simpsons or Eatons department store. No, it was Simpsons. No matter. Its location was less important than the dangerously thrilling ride on the sloped wooden slats. They showed no mercy for the unprepared or the unaware as they continued to roll up, up, up in perpetual motion. You had to choose when to step on and take hold of the moving handrail and indecision was met with great impatience from the Torontonians piling up behind you. The steps rumbled and rolled beneath your feet as though they would come apart at any given moment. And the ride up was nothing compared to the courage required for the ride down. We loved it, Jaynie and I. Mom, of course, was quite cosmopolitan about it all, having lived in Toronto as a young woman and being familiar with city life.

We never bought anything during these escalator adventures. We just walked around the huge stores and looked at things until it was time to retrieve our suitcase from the bus station and head back to the subway. Down the steps, into the rush of wind as a train roared into the underground station squealing its brakes. It's here! No, too late. It's gone. Drop the slim token in the slot and push the metal turnstile with all your might. Stand back near the white tiled wall where QUEEN was painted in bold black letters. Wait for the next train. Another rush of wind. Another train. Hold hands. The crowd of people moves forward and as the doors of the train slide open everyone pushes in. Mom pulls us forward and finds a seat that the three of us can share. We're off! It's a short ride but a wonderful one, nonetheless. A stop or two later and we arrive.

Now at Union Station, we'll wait on the long, highly polished wooden benches until boarding is announced. Jayne and I sit together while Mom goes into the tuck shop and purchases three cheese sandwiches that will be our supper on the train.

"Platform three southbound train now boarding for Port Credit, Hamilton, Grimsby, St. Catharines, Welland, Port Colborne, Fort Erie, and Buffalo. All aboard, please."

Our trip to Toronto was done. The Santa Claus Parade was over. The bagpipes, subway, and cafeteria Jell-O would be pasted into our memory books, each of us colouring the pages according to our own personal remembrances.

A month later, Jayne and I woke to the silent, glistening, snow-covered world of Christmas morning. At the foot of our four-poster bed were two lumpy, white socks tied to the foot board and bursting with treats! First out of the sock was the candy cane. Now a colouring book rolled up in an elastic band. Crayons! A chocolate treat wrapped in coloured foil to look like Santa. And the annual mandarin orange with loose hard candies in the sock toe. There, on our bed, we would colour and snack until Mom called to tell us it was time to come downstairs. Hands on the banister we ran down the steps, Jayne first, past the living room and into the dining room where our tall Christmas tree stood in the bay window, fully lit and sparkling with tinsel.

We each had a side of the tree where our gifts would be waiting. This side was for Jayne. Next to that and in the front of the tree were Jim's then Paul's gifts. And mine were on the other side of the tree.

As we ran into the dining room, we saw it. A walking doll! Standing there with Jayne's gifts. She was beautiful. She had light brown hair, a blue cotton dress, and white socks and shoes! Our Christmas wish came true.

"Pooh!" my sister called. "Look, we got our walking doll!" I laughed and we hugged.

Then Dad says to me, "Don't you want to see what Santa brought for you, Pooh?"

Yes! I ran around to my side of the tree and stopped in my tracks. There, standing all on her own was another walking doll. Blonde, beautiful in the same dress as Jayne's doll but pink. Two. Two walking dolls. How did they know? How did Santa tell them?

"Jaynie! Look!"

Holding my treasure in my arms I walked around the tree to show Jayne. She was holding her doll by the hand and leading it forward in its first steps. She gasped. We giggled. We walked our dolls. Behind our play, we hear Dad laugh. Mom is crying.

* * *

Paul is in the dining room on the phone with Mom. I don't know where she is, but Dad is at work.

"Just a minute, Mom. I'll check."

He puts down the receiver and runs to the front living room window. Rain is pouring off the front porch roof like a waterfall. There is a huge crack of thunder, and he runs back to the phone.

"No, it's all right. It's still standing. No, that was thunder. I'm sure, Mom. The one that's leaning? It's still standing."

Another boom of thunder.

"Jayne, Winnifred, go into the kitchen. Just go there and wait for me."

Jayne wants to know what's going on.

"Why, Paul? What's wrong?"

"Just go stand by the kitchen door."

So, we do. But we can still hear him on the phone to Mom, raising his voice now to be heard above the storm.

"Lots of water, yes. But I don't think it's from the river. Okay. Will you call them? Say we're coming? As soon as it lets up a bit. Okay. I will. Okay. Bye."

He hangs up the phone and comes into the kitchen.

"Okay. Come out onto the porch with me. We have to make a run for it up to Dixon's house. We'll wait for it to let up a bit."

He opens the kitchen door, and we step out onto the back porch. The rain is a solid sheet so thick you can barely see Rumley's house across the street. There's another deafening boom of thunder.

Jayne is apprehensive. "I don't want to go out there. Let's just wait here at home."

"We can't," Paul answers. "Mom is afraid that the big tree out front might fall and hit the house. You don't want to be here if that happens, do you?"

We stand, Jayne and me, hand in hand, and wait. But nothing changes. The rain is endless, relentless. The street is a river. Now the wind has picked up and is pushing water onto the back porch. Our feet are soaked. Suddenly, a deafening boom and we feel the porch shudder under our feet as though the whole house has shaken.

"Damn!" Paul grabs us each by a hand and yells. "Okay! Let's go!"

There is no choice in the matter. He has a tight hold on each of us and we are suddenly out in the middle of the storm. Then he pushes us forward.

"Run! Run to Dixon's!"

"Where are you going?"

Paul has turned back and is running to our house. "Just go! I'll be right behind you."

Jayne grabs my hand and pulls me up Almond Street and onto Dixon's porch. Mrs. Dixon is waiting at her front door for us with a towel and tells us to take off our wet shoes because she's just washed the floor. But where is Paul? Where is he?

Mrs. Dixon leads us into her kitchen and has us stand by the radiator. It's warm. Now there is a knocking at the door, and she opens it for Paul.

"Take off your wet shoes," is her greeting.

"May I call my mom, please? I just want to tell her that the girls are okay."

"I suppose."

Again, we hear his side of the conversation.

"No, it didn't fall. I don't know. Yes, I ran back to check but the house is okay. Something fell but it wasn't that tree. I don't know. Yes. Yes, they're here. Okay.

He hands Mrs. Dixon the receiver and walks into the kitchen where Jayne and I are leaning against the radiator.

"Okay?" He smiles at us.

"We're okay." Jayne answers for us both.

Years later Mom would tell me that she had called Dad at work to say she was worried about the storm. During Hurricane Hazel in 1954 there were 35 people killed in Toronto when the Humber River burst its banks. Our house was only a road away from the Welland River. But this was not Hurricane Hazel.

One of the large evergreens that graced our front yard leaned dangerously toward the house. What if it fell and crashed through the roof? Apparently, Dad said he wished it would. They could use the insurance money. I don't know if that was true. Maybe he was just tired. Very sick and very tired. And he hated that house on River Road.

Hours later, when the storm passed, we made our way home again. Paul went out onto the front porch just to check on the leaning tree. It leaned there still. Further along the front yard, however, another tree was missing. Another evergreen, which was never suspect, had fallen straight back between the hedges beside the house, crashed into the backyard, landing between our swing set and the sand box and coming to rest just a few feet short of the garage. Mom always called that a miracle. She said that the Lord had saved our home.

The giant tree lay across our yard for a day or two. Ours was not the only property to have lost a tree in that storm and there was no shortage of men with chainsaws prepared to haul these trees away for a price. That was not an option for us. But neither was it an option for our dad to do the work. When he wasn't at work he was resting.

On the Saturday after the storm Jayne is looking out our bedroom window at the major activity in our yard.

"Come look at this."

People are gathered around the fallen tree. Jim, Paul, their friends, and our neighbours were organizing themselves into work groups, saws in hand, to cut up and haul away the fallen tree for Herb Bray. What excitement! It looked like the whole neighbourhood was there including Locky Fowler and Stan Ryan from up the street, Fred Rumley from across the street, and that really cute friend of Jim's.

"Let's get dressed and go outside with everyone!" my sister says.

Jayne and I both had a childish crush on that really cute friend of Jim's. Just as we were about to run down the stairs, we met Mom coming up.

"Where are you girls going?"

"Outside to help."

"No. There's nothing you can do out there. You will only be in the way. Come on. Back to your room."

"But we can help. We can work." Jayne answers definitively.

"If you want to work, stay here and clean up this bedroom."

Ugh. The impossible task. We had never been able to clean our room to anyone's satisfaction. With no closet and no toy box where were we supposed to put everything? But back to our room we trudged with Mom following close behind.

"Just pick up all your clothes and put them on the bed. Then sort the toys from the books and put them neatly against the wall. Come on then."

She supervises, briefly, as we grudgingly start the chore. Then she leaves.

"This is impossible." Jayne complains. She drops an armful of clothing and goes back to the window. I join her.

"Everybody else is outside," I say.

"I know." She is angry. "This isn't fair. It's going to take us all day."

Then her eyes sparkle with conspiracy. "Let's just shove everything under the bed and go out."

"Okay." That seemed like a good idea to me.

Within minutes our room looked quite tidy. Somewhat devoid of toys, clothes, and books, but tidy, nonetheless.

"Let's go!"

My sister leads the way down the stairs and out the front door. Almost immediately someone shows us where we can stand to be out of the way. But to be that close to the fallen tree was almost irresistible. You could actually touch the pine needles and cones that, until the storm, had hung so high above the yard. And the whole yard smelled like a Christmas tree. The sawing, heaving, and hauling continued.

"Hey, look!" someone calls. "A bird's nest!"

Really? A real bird's nest? Yes. There was even a small blue egg in it. That would be something to have.

"Hey, Jim. Can I have this for my girlfriend?" Pete wanted to know.

"Sure." our brother tells him.

Jayne and I begin our own search near the top of the tree that is laying near our sandbox. There must be other bird's nests. And there are. But we don't find them.

"Here's another one! Hey, Stan. Catch!" Someone hurls the nest at Stan and the small treasure explodes against his back.

"Knock it off!" someone else hollers.

Jayne and I keep looking but can't really get close to the trunk because the branches scratch our legs and arms. Our search is earnest but not very productive. And when frustration wins out over ambition I drop to the ground and begin to cry.

"Hey, Paul. Your kid sister is crying."

Paul stops what he's doing and comes over to check on us.

"What's the matter?" he asks, softly.

"She wanted a bird's nest." Jayne tells him.

"Oh. I don't think there are any more than two or three in a tree." he explains.

"It's not fair! It's our tree." I sob at the injustice.

"I know." He strokes my head. "How about if I keep looking for you? Maybe I'll find one more."

"Really?"

"Really." He smiles down at me.

"Okay," I sniff.

"What are you two doing out here?" Uh oh. Mom must have heard my sobbing and now she is marching across the yard.

"I told you to clean your bedroom."

Jayne protests. "We did."

"You did not! Now get back into the house and upstairs."

She takes each of us by the hand and drags us back into the front yard, past all the neighbours and friends, to the front porch. Then one at a time she smacks our bums and sends us up the steps. Right in front of everyone. Right in front of Jim's really cute friend.

It's no use. She has discovered our stash under the bed and has dragged it all back out again.

"Now do as you're told and clean this room." She leaves, closing the door behind her.

What's the point? Together we sit on our bed. I sulk. Jayne fumes. After a time, she slides off the bed and stands in the middle of the room.

"We better do something, I guess. You line up the toys. I'll stack the books."

"Okay."

Eventually, the late Saturday afternoon sun pours in our front bedroom window. It must be getting near dinner time. Out the window we see piles of logs and evergreen branches, some people still sawing, others sitting on the grass and drinking water or coffee from tall thermoses. What a waste of a day.

Now Mom calls, "You girls can come down now."

We don't need a second invitation. Down the stairs and out the front door again. We round the house and head into the backyard where the top of the tree used to lay. It's all chopped up and piled throughout the yard. No hope of ever finding a bird's nest now.

Jayne and I sit on our swings. My feet dangle above the grass. I have no heart to pump.

"Don't cry, Pooh." my sister consoles.

Then Paul comes over to us. He has something cupped in his hands.

"Here you go." He hands me a small bird's nest. It's perfect.

"For me?"

"For you to share."

"Is there an egg?" I ask.

"Oh! She wants an egg, too. No. No egg. Just the nest." Our brother smiles.

"Oh, thank you, thank you, thank you! Look, Jaynie! Paul found us a nest."

"Wow. Thanks."

We fuss over the gift and, together, carry it around to the back porch where we can sit and decide where it should live. We never notice that our brother's hands are caked with mud and bits of dry grass.

*   *   *

Jim was sixteen now. Old enough to smoke, but not around his mother. Sometimes he'd sneak one with Dad. Export A. He was old enough to date Betty, too, the pretty girl who lived just up the street. And old enough to quit school as had been suggested to him by the high school vice-principal.

"You are obviously not interested in education," he'd been told. "You should just leave."

"With pleasure," he thought. "And screw you, too, old man."

What did he know about it, anyway? Nothing, the old coot.

Quitting had never been Jim's plan. There had never really been a plan, come to think of it, until recently. His grades had been good in previous years. He liked to read. He liked to draw. He liked to argue his point too. But that had all been before. Every day now for the last two years or so the long walk from the house on River Road to Welland High School had gotten longer, harder, and less easy to bear. Every morning he wondered what the day would bring.

Dread. It would bring dread. Would he be late again and be grilled by the vice-principal? That happened mostly in winter. The long walk was harder in winter. But he was tough, he told his pals. Who needed boots? So, what if I'm late? Would the English teacher notice that his essay wasn't finished? Or maybe he'd use his work as an example of how essays were to be written in ink, not pencil like his. What if someone noticed the tear in his shirt sleeve? Just roll the cuffs up. To hell with proper attire rules. Old Man Coot wouldn't like that. Mom had given him fifty cents for lunch from the cafeteria, because he would not carry an old metal lunch pail. Not a chance. But then again, maybe his stomach wouldn't wait until lunchtime and would growl during math class again.

To hell with it. Who cared anyway? He'd stop at Kiraly's store and get a pack of smokes with the lunch money. That would keep the hunger down. Missing school no longer mattered because Jim had a plan that not even Dad knew about.

Sometimes when Dad was working four to twelve, he would go visit him at the plant during his lunch break. They'd sit side by side, leaning against the outside brick wall of the old drop forge factory, sharing a smoke, talking, and not talking. They were both men of few words.

More recently, though, Dad would ask how school was. Jim's evasive answer would prompt concern in his father's eyes, and he would say,

"School is important, Son. You don't want to work in a factory like this all your life, do you?"

No. Jim knew he would never spend his life doing that, working everyday inside a hot and noisy plant of any kind. But he also knew he didn't need High School, either. Because Jim had a plan.

*   *   *

Up the street and around two corners on Oxford Road lived Mom's friend, Mrs. Nix. Her name was Lola, but of course, we called her Mrs. Nix. She and her husband, Emerson, and their teenage daughter, Gay, had a small narrow bungalow that faced the fields of Cullimore's farm on the other side of Oxford Road. Mrs. Nix's mother used to live with them. She had the middle bedroom and slept in a narrow, single bed. But the old woman was gone now so that bedroom sat empty.

Along the side of their house was a vegetable garden that produced beets, peas, spinach, and potatoes. There was always food at

Mrs. Nix's. She was a good friend to our mom for lots of reasons. But my memory of her is of pots and pots of tea brewed on the wood stove, which was one of the sources of heat in the little house. It was also the means by which bathwater was boiled in an enamel pan. There was no tub or shower. Only a kind of indoor outhouse at the back door that didn't flush. But the linoleum floors always gleamed, the tea towels were crisp and clean, and no dust lived anywhere in Mrs. Nix's house.

Often, when Mom took Jayne and I to visit Mrs. Nix, we would stay for dinner. I think that was probably Mom's hope and intention, especially if Dad was working four to twelve. Jayne and I were unaware of that. We just knew that there would be pots and pots of tea, homemade pickled beets, and creamed peas.

Because Jayne and I had very long hair, Gay Nix used to play with it, combing, styling, and fashioning it into the latest look. That was usually an acceptable activity until the day Mom and I went to visit, and Gay decided to give me a beehive.

She teased and backcombed my long hair, then pushed it up on top of my small head, poked it full of bobby pins, and smothered me in hairspray. The finishing touch was a gold and rhinestone barrette shaped like a leaf and clipped onto the side of my head. She handed me the mirror. It was beautiful. I thought you had to be a teenager to have this kind of hairstyle. I wasn't a teenager. Far from it. But Gay seemed very pleased with herself and with my reaction, and she handed me a stick of Doublemint gum.

We sat in her room, playing her 45s very loudly. "Please Please Me." "Love Me Do." "P.S. I Love You". Over and over again. Gay was a big Beatles fan. But then, who wasn't? We listened to other records too. "Blue on Blue," "It's My Party" and "My Boyfriend's Back." But we always came back to the Beatles. We filled the afternoon with loud music, nail polish, lipstick, and gum and I soon forgot about my hair.

Mom and Mrs. Nix sat at the kitchen table the whole time, talking. By what must have been their third pot of tea, Mom called to me that it was time to go. I walked into the kitchen.

"Good Lord! What have you done?"

That wasn't exactly the reaction I expected. Mom was horrified.

"What have you done to your hair?"

"It's a beehive." I loved it.

Mrs. Nix shouted to her daughter. "Gay! Gay! Come here. I mean it!"

You had to shout to Gay because she was almost completely deaf and had been all her life. Because she had never been given a hearing aid or any other kind of help, her speech was thick and inarticulate. Conveniently for her, however, there were times when she was more deaf than others.

"Gay! I know you can hear me. Come here! I mean it, now! What did you do?'

Gay stepped around the corner into the kitchen and smiled. "Wha . . .?"

"Oh, my Lord." Mom is nearly frantic. "How am I ever going to get this out?"

She's already pulling at my hair.

"Ow! Ow!"

"I'll never get this untangled." Mom sounds as though she is about to cry.

Mrs. Nix is still shouting at Gay. "She's just a little girl! What did you do?"

Gay rolls her eyes. "Wha- Wha's a madder?"

"You comb that out! Come on, comb it out right now! Now I mean it!" Mrs. Nix yells.

Mom is still tugging at me.

"Ow! Ow! Mommy, stop!" It hurts, but I don't want to cry.

"Oh, it's no use. What a mess."

Gay has turned with a shrug and left the fuss in the kitchen. "Please Please Me" blares from her room.

"Turn that down. Gay! You're gonna get it! Turn that down. Now I mean it! Oh, she doesn't hear me."

Gay never hears her mother no matter how much she means it. Gay never "gets it" either.

The next morning, I sat in the dining room as Mom tried to pull a comb through the rat's nest that was my hair. She had given up on it last night and sent me to bed in a mess of knots and a puddle of tears. But today I have to go to school, and I can't go looking like this. The bell will ring soon. Jayne has already left for school. Panic builds in my chest. I'll be late! I'll be late for school and everyone will stare at me.

"Mommy, please. Let me go."

"You cannot go looking like that! What were you thinking?"

"Ow. Ow. OW!"

She's taking her frustration and anger out on my head. She throws down the comb. "It's useless! You'll have to go like this. I don't know what else to do besides cut it."

"No! Don't cut my hair. Don't cut my hair!"

Then Dad emerges from his bedroom, just off the dining room.

"Who's this? Little Punkinhead?"

"Daddy! Don't cut my hair."

"No one's going to cut your hair, Pooh. Give me the comb, Cathy."

She hands him her comb. "It's useless. And look at the time. I'll be late."

"You go on ahead. I'll take care of her."

"You're supposed to be resting."

"Just go. I'll get her off to school."

"Thank you." She's gone.

My father pulls up the kitchen stool and sits behind me, comb in hand. He takes hold of the thick lock of knotted hair at the back of my head and begins to gently pull it apart. Just then we hear the school bell ring.

"Oh no! Daddy. I have to go."

"Not until we get this sorted out."

"But I'm late for school."

"You may be late, but no child of mine is going anywhere looking like this. You'll go when we're done."

I don't remember how long it took him to comb out my hair. I do remember him talking to himself under his breath. How could anyone let this happen? Stupid people. Just a child, etc. I also remember that he wasn't angry with me. He didn't know how to braid my hair when he was done. The knots were gone, but all my hair frizzed out around my head like a dried out scarecrow. Still, he did know how to calm my fears about being late for school.

"I'll tell them it was my fault. Don't worry about it." And I believed him because he was my dad.

I still hated being late. People still stared at me when I finally walked into class. But it wasn't because I was a Punkinhead. My dad made sure of that.

*   *   *

It's an old habit my sister has. She doesn't really have to look at her hands anymore to tell left from right. But old habits die hard. And this habit was born hard on a hot summer's day on King Street in 1962.

When our dad is on night shift, it's best if we leave him in peace to sleep through the day, especially in the summer. Rest is often hard won for him. So on this particular day Mom, Jayne, and I head out to spend the afternoon at Merritt Park.

Despite the temperature we keep a good pace as we walk up River Road, down Main Street, and on to Merritt Park to find Mom's favourite spot under a tree by the canal. She settles on the grass with a book while Jayne and I slide down the canal bank to sit on a flat rock and dip our feet in the cool water. No boats in sight yet but there are sure to be one or two as the day wears on.

The large, round, cement water fountain in the middle of the park is a good place to cool down as well. It looks very much like a layer cake. A big, green layer cake. Streams of water shoot up from the sides and into the centre as more water cascades down the middle, flowing and splashing and spraying our hot faces. Our cotton tops are wet but not quite enough to cool us down entirely. We head back to where Mom has retreated into the world of her book so totally that she is seemingly transported to a cooler land. Calm, cool, and content. We plop down beside her.

Jayne has no compunction about interrupting Mom's reverie.

"Mommy, we're thirsty and the drinking fountain isn't working."

"Oh?" Our mother looks up from her book. "Well, would you like a cold pop?"

"Yes, please!" we answer in unison.

She opens her purse and takes out two nickels, one for each of us.

"Go on up to Bitando's and get yourselves each a pop." She hands the money to Jayne.

"Thank you!" we gush.

Bitando's store is just up the street from the park. Not far at all. We'll walk through the park and past the big green and white Welland Club. We head off together as Mom calls out, "Hold hands and stay together."

"Okay!"

At the end of the park, we step out onto the hot sidewalk, hand in hand, avoiding the cracks that will "break your mother's back." Jumping over the parts where the sidewalk has heaved, we pass the few houses on this side of King Street. One of the houses has a long, low porch where two old men sit in the shade and watch us go by. They don't say anything. They just watch.

Up the step and through the beaded curtains into Bitando's store, we step into a cooler world where a fan whirls above and cold pop lives in a deep metal case filled with chilled water.

"Let's get red pop." I say to my sister.

"Or maybe Orange Crush." she replies. "Or maybe one red pop and one Orange Crush."

"And we'll share." I suggest.

It's decided. Jayne lifts the metal lid on the pop case and pulls out two cold, wet, glass bottles of summer relief. At the counter, she puts down the two nickels, and then we take turns at the bottle opener at the front of the pop case. One long swig each and switch. Another long swig each and we switch again. Time to head back to Mom and the park.

The walk back from Bitando's is somewhat cooler now that we're refreshed. Our glass pop bottles are cold and wet and feel good when we rub them against our cheeks.

We're going to pass the two old men on the porch again. I don't like the way they just sit there so I suggest, "Come on. Let's run!" And we're off.

I take the lead and almost immediately pass by the long, old-man porch. Then I hear Jayne cry out. I stop and turn. She's sitting on the sidewalk crying.

"Jaynie!" I yell and run back to her. She doesn't answer. She just sits there crying. She's holding the top half of her Orange Crush bottle. The jagged bottom half lays in front of her where it has rolled down the heave in the sidewalk. Her hand is covered in blood.

"Jaynie!" I cry, plopping down beside her. What do I do? I don't know what to do!

But all Jayne can manage is, "Mommy."

I have to get Mommy. I stand to run back to the park and get Mommy. But here she is now, running toward us. Someone in the park has heard the commotion and sent her flying up King Street.

"My God! What happened?" She is kneeling next to Jayne now and holding her bleeding hand. But Jayne can't answer. She just cries and shakes.

"Take her to the clinic up the street. She'll need stitches." A woman I don't know is standing behind me. Maybe she's the one who alerted our mother. Stitches? What are stitches?

"It's a vaccination clinic." Mom says.

"But the doctor will be there. He can give you first aid," the woman replies.

"Yes. Yes. That's best."

Mom has wrapped Jayne's hand with a cloth that has magically appeared. Perhaps it's a hanky.

"What happened, Honey?" she asks Jayne, who sobs, "I tripped."

Jayne is standing now, leaning against Mom and dripping blood down both of them.

"Dear God," Mom whispers. Then she sees the two old men sitting on the porch and asks them, "What happened? Did you see what happened?"

But the old men don't say anything. They don't do anything. They just watch.

The clinic. I know this place. I remember being here with Mom. We had lined up with lots of other kids and their parents to get into the building. The little boy behind me was crying and pleading with his mother. He was scared, nearly terrified. I was curious why. I had no idea what we were there for. But his mother pointed to me and said to her son, "You see, this little girl isn't crying. You're not afraid, are you dear?"

I shake my head "no."

"See?" she continues. "If this little girl isn't afraid, you shouldn't be either. You're a boy!"

Soon enough though, I was to discover that the only reason I wasn't afraid was because I didn't know they were going shove a needle in my arm. Polio vaccine. That's why I know this place.

I don't want to leave her side. I stand by the bed in the small vaccination clinic where my sister lies, her left arm outstretched, palm side up. The doctor and the nurse have cleaned the blood away but when they gently pull the piece of glass from her hand Jaynie whimpers and Mom nearly faints.

"Sit down, Mrs. Bray," the nurse tells her, leading her to a chair. But I will not leave my sister's side.

Now the doctor and nurse confer then turn to Mom.

"She will need stitches, Mrs. Bray. Just two or three. I can do it here as a first aid measure, but we don't have any anesthetic in this clinic for such a procedure. Can you drive her to Emergency?"

"No. No, I don't have the car."

"Can you call your husband?"

"No! Oh, no. He's sleeping. Night shift. No, I mustn't."

The doctor and the nurse confer again. Then, needing confirmation, the doctor says to our mom.

"The wound needs to be stitched or it will not heal properly and could become infected. Do you want me to proceed, then?"

"Yes. If you must." Mom holds her head in her hands.

"All right." Then the doctor says to the nurse, "Let's get this done."

Now the nurse gently takes Jayne's other hand and smiles down at her.

"Sweetie, the doctor is going to fix your hand and close the wound. It's going to sting a little, but you just hold my hand and squeeze really hard if it hurts. Look at me. You don't have to watch him. And you can cry if you want to. It won't take long, Sweetie. I promise."

Jayne sniffs. "Okay."

Now the doctor steps in front of me. Pulling a white metal tray on a wheeled table with him he fusses with some items that I can't see but eventually takes Jayne's hand gently in his. The next thing he does I *can* see. It's a needle and a thread. A shiny needle and black thread and he sticks it into the palm of my sister's hand and begins to sew. She whimpers. The nurse strokes her head. He stitches again. I can't believe what I'm seeing. He's sewing up my sister.

"Oh Jaynie!" I cry. "Stop it! You're hurting her!"

The doctor only now becomes aware of me standing behind him. He stops and looks at the nurse.

"Mrs. Bray, perhaps you could take your other little girl outside to wait," she suggests.

But Mom doesn't hear. She is sitting on the chair against the wall, still holding her head in her hands. She's praying.

"Mrs. Bray?" No answer. "Honey, go sit with your mommy," the nurse says to me.

"I want to stay with Jaynie."

"It's okay, Pooh. It doesn't hurt." Probably the only lie my sister ever told me.

"It doesn't?"

"No. Go sit with Mommy. Don't watch. I don't want you to watch."

"Okay." I sit next to our mother who looks over and takes hold of me. She squeezes me too tightly. "It's okay," I tell her, "Jaynie says it doesn't hurt." She squeezes me again.

Three or four stitches? I don't know. But it doesn't take long. And the kind nurse never leaves her side. When they finish, the doctor and the nurse gush with praise at what a good and brave little girl she is.

"Here, Honey," the nurse says as she hands Jayne a small pill and a drink of water from a tiny paper cup.

Then the doctor begins to wrap Jayne's hand with white gauze. He asks Mom, "Do you have a ride home? She shouldn't jostle this hand for a while."

"No," Mom answers. I recognize her tone. It's something like embarrassment. "No, we walked."

"Your husband—"

"He's sleeping. He can't be disturbed. We'll walk."

"Where do you live?" the doctor wants to know.

"Down River Road" is all Mom will say.

The doctor and the nurse confer silently this time. She hands him more gauze bandaging and by the time they finish with Jayne's hand it looks like a huge white cast wrapped up past her wrist. As they help Jayne down from the table the doctor gives Mom her instructions.

"We've given her Aspirin, but she will need more in a few hours. Keep the dressing dry and as immobile as possible for at least twenty-four hours. And you should take her to your own doctor to have the bandage removed and the wound checked for infection. She won't be able to use this hand for a while."

"Yes. Thank you." And we leave.

As we walk along River Road on our way home, I look behind me whenever I hear a car coming. Sometimes when the three of us are walking River Road a friendly neighbour will stop and pick us up to give us a ride home, especially if it's raining. Or snowing and cold. This would be a good day for a friendly neighbour because the walk seems longer than usual. But no such luck on this hot summer's day. Jayne holds her left hand in the crook of her right arm and every once in a while she sniffs. She's walking slowly with Mom on one side of her and me on the other. Another car. A friendly wave, but that's all. By the time we get home, Jayne is spent.

We step into the kitchen through the back door and Mom whispers, "Hush now. Daddy is sleeping." Except that he is not.

"It's all right," he says as he steps out of their bedroom and into the kitchen. "It's too hot to sleep. You're home early."

And then he sees Jayne. "What the hell? What happened to my little girl?"

That is all it takes. Jayne's pent-up anguish bursts forth as she runs to our dad, dissolving into tears. He crouches down to hold her, and she sobs into his embrace.

Mom's voice quivers. "It's not as bad as it looks. She's all right, really."

"All right? She's come home in a cast!" He seems angry and distraught in equal portions.

"I send her out for day of fun and you bring her home in a cast."

"Oh, Herb." Mom sinks into a chair.

"What happened, Honey?" Dad asks Jayne.

"I tripped. With a pop bottle. I was running." She snuggles into his neck breathing in his warmth.

"Okay. It's okay. Come sit with Daddy." Dad carries her into the living room and settles them both into his La-Z-Boy chair where he rocks her and hums comfort.

When Dr. White removes the bandages, he comments on the stitches.

"They've done a good job of first aid," he tells our mother. "But it's a quickly done job to be sure. Looks like it will scar. Bring her back in a week or so and I'll take the stitches out. We'll know better then."

In 1962 my sister earned her first battle scar. In the years to come she would press it into service to help her know left from right, a confusion thrust upon her by an educational system that refused to let her be left-handed. I see her now, telling me which side of the street we need to walk to find that very cool vintage shop.

"It's on the left side, I think." She looks at her hand and the ancient scar out of habit. "Nope," she says. "Wrong one. That's right."

*   *   *

Jim saw the car pull into the driveway at the side of the house. He didn't recognize the vehicle as being Dr. White's. Besides, Dad was sleeping and not expecting a house call. But when the uniformed man got out of the car Jim had no doubt who it was. What was he doing here? He walked away and into the dining room just as there was a knock at the side kitchen door.

"Oh, who's that now?" Mom whispered as she came out of the bedroom, closing the door behind her softly.

"Don't know," Jim answered, still walking away from the kitchen.

Mom opened the door to see a tall, uniformed man filling the doorway. "Mrs. Bray?"

"Yes."

"I'm Captain William Swayze, Canadian Armed Forces Reserve."

"How can I help you, Captain?"

"I am here on a matter concerning your son, Jim."

"My son? Well, you'd better come in."

"Thank you."

"Do you mind if we stay here in the kitchen? My husband is sleeping in the next room."

"Yes, of course. Thank you."

She offered him a seat and they sat at the kitchen table.

"I understand that Jim was a member of the Cadet Corp for some time until recently," the Captain said.

"Yes," Mom answered, not masking a certain pride. "Both our boys were Cadets."

"Is he at home?"

"Yes." Mom walked to the dining room where Jim stood looking out the bay window and told him to come into the kitchen.

There was no avoiding it now. He walked into the kitchen and Captain Swayze stood to face him.

"Hello, Jim. Good to meet you."

"And you, Sir."

Jim remained standing just a few steps away, but the Captain sat back down and said to Mom, "I'm here to follow up on Jim's recent visit to the Lake Street Armory in St. Catharines a short while ago."

Mom turned to Jim. "When did you go to St. Catharines?"

"A while ago," he answered, not to his mother's satisfaction.

The Captain continued. "The reason for my visit is this: I want to encourage you to remain in school, Jim, and graduate. It is possible for you to enlist now, of course, but with a high school diploma you would be an excellent candidate for the Regular Officer Training Program. But you need to finish high school first."

"I don't know what you mean, Captain," Mom said, evenly. "Jim is not quitting school. Wherever would you get such an idea?"

Assessing the situation, Captain Swayze looked at Jim and asked, "Son, have you not spoken to your parents about this matter?" He looked at Jim, waiting for a reply but none came. So, he spoke on his behalf.

"Mrs. Bray, he has already done so."

"Done what?" Mom asked.

"Quit school."

"What?" Mom blanched as the blood ran from her face. She dropped her head into her hands and cradled it there.

"Oh, my dear Lord," she murmured. "What were you thinking? Your father will have a fit."

Speaking directly to Jim, the Captain said, "It's not too late to re-enroll."

"No sir," Jim said, evenly. "I'm sorry, Sir, but no. I want to enlist. I want to go into the Service now."

"That is your choice, of course, but you know you are too young. You will need your parents' permission."

No one spoke for what seemed to Jim an eternity, so he finally broke the silence.

"Mom?"

"What is it?"

"Will you sign for me so I can go into the Service? Into the Armed Forces."

She lifted her head and looked directly at her eldest son.

"The Armed Forces! Absolutely not. What are you thinking? You have to go back to school."

Jim's blood churned with frustration. He looked to the captain and then to Mom.

"Then I'll get a job until I'm old enough to sign myself up. But I'm not going back to school."

Now that it had been said out loud, he knew it to be true. And in that moment Jim saw his plan unravel and his entire future change.

*   *   *

The last day of school we were handed our final report cards, safely sealed in brown envelopes, and entrusted to us to carry home to our parents. The final dismissal bell rang and the yard at Riverview School exploded with children bursting with energy and the wild anticipation of throwing off our shoes for the summer. Jayne and I met on the front lawn of the school and ran home together, hand in hand. Liberation! Flying through the front door, we kicked off our shoes, ran through the dining room, dropped our envelopes on the table and headed to the backyard where we would swing away the chalk dust of the past school year. That was, until Dad came home from work, and we were summoned back into the dining room for the great reveal. Our final reports. Jayne and I stood together while our parents sat at the table, two brown envelopes between them. Mom opened mine first and read aloud.

"Polite, well behaved, participates in class. All satisfactory. Good. Now, grades. Reading, spelling, writing, all A's. Arithmetic C. That's disappointing. What happened there?"

My face burned.

"Sorry."

I don't tell them it's the flash cards. I hate those flash cards. They make me panic and I forget the answers. Then everyone stares when I get the answers wrong, and I forget everything.

"Well, you'll have to try harder next year." Then she reads, "Winnifred has been promoted to Grade Two. Good."

Mom reaches for Jayne's report card, but Dad takes it from her.

"Let's see," he says.

But he doesn't read the grades. Instead, he smiles up at Jayne and says,

"Jayne has been promoted to Grade Three."

"Really Daddy?" my sister gasps. "Really?"

"Really," he says as he puts the report back into its envelope. "Well I think this deserves celebration. A reward for both of you for passing. What do you say to bicycles?"

We don't know what to say, it's such a surprise. Nevertheless, within two weeks we each had our own bicycle. Identical chrome and blue three-speed bikes delivered by Simpson Sears right to our back door. Identical except that one had a small chrome piece on the front fender, and one did not. That was how we would tell them apart.

The next order of business was learning to ride. Jayne was a natural and with Dad's help was soon gliding up and down Almond Street and River Road, glowing with newfound freedom. I required a bit more instruction and courage.

On the sidewalk in front of our house my first step was to stand astride my new bike. According to my Dad it was just the right size for me. He held the bike steady while I put a foot on one pedal and lifted myself into the seat.

"There. That wasn't so hard," he said, smiling. "Now, I'll hold the back of the seat and you put your other foot on the pedal."

Before I knew it, I was on the bike and we were rolling forward with my dad's constant encouragement.

"If you feel yourself tipping just turn into the fall and face it. And you will get your balance back. Now pedal! Keep pedalling. Push yourself forward. Your momentum will keep you from falling."

I could hear him talking behind me. His hand on the seat.

"I've got you. I won't let you fall."

From the sidewalk in front of our house to the walk in front of the school, my dad held me steady.

"That's it. Keep pedalling." His breath sounded short-winded. I saw the hill coming up.

"Daddy, stop! The hill!"

"You're okay," he called. "Keep going. You are doing it on your own."

And I realized that he was no longer there holding the back of my bicycle seat. A sudden thrill of freedom washed over me, and I flew down the hill, leaving my dad far behind. But his words stayed with me —always. If you feel yourself tipping, turn into the fall, face it and you will get your balance back. Just keep pedalling.

*　*　*

I open the letter from my sister. There are several photos and a short letter, printed in dot matrix on pink paper and double-spaced for exclamation.

Isn't IT Beautiful!!!!!???

The photos don't really do it justice. The painting is so detailed! It really is a work of art. If you look hard, you can see the shadow of the porch light (Towards the mailbox and doorbell.) It's like that all the way around. The shadows are in perspective. None of the shrubs are the same. Each little brick, slat in the shutters and railing post. Is perfect! The roof is slate! Randal is making a door for me at work. On the inside shot, you can really see the detail in the roof. Sorry, you can't see much of the last room. That's the one I told you has the robin painted outside the window. There are plants on both mantles and on corner nooks in the kitchen. Doesn't it bring back a lot of memories? Wish you could see it for yourself.

I LOVE this doll house as much as I did the first time. Hey, Pooh! I feel like, only two men in my whole life have really loved me for who I am. And they both bought me the same Doll House! Ain't life grand ???!!!
YOUR ONE AND ONLY

The arrival of the Simpson Sears Christmas catalogue had always signalled the beginning of the "Wish Season." Jayne and I sat on the living room rug, each with a pen in hand, ready to circle the things we hoped Santa would bring. You had to dog-ear the page, too, so that Mom and Dad would know what pages to turn to.

There were so many things to look at on the girls' pages. We didn't care about the cowboy hats, cap guns, and train sets on the boys' pages. Paul liked the Mr. Potato Head pieces that you could stick into real potatoes and watch his face shrivel over time. But Jayne and I poured over pictures of toy dish sets, dolls that talked, cried, and laughed, telephones, cash registers and typewriters that really worked. I really hoped for a Slinky and circled that picture twice.

There were things we passed over because they were too big to ask for. Things like the electric toy car that you could actually get into and really drive. Or the pink toy kitchen "complete with fridge, stove, sink, oven and pantry, all of steel and just her size." Paul read the ad to us. You could get a washing machine too. We didn't circle any of that. The toy doctor's bag was black. The nurse's bag was red. And roller skates came complete with two keys in case you lost one.

Jayne turned the page and pointed. Her eyes grew round like saucers. "Look!"

"What is it?" I moved closer to her to see what she was looking at.

"A doll house. Oh, look at it." She showed me the catalogue page.

"No, that's a real house." I tell her.

"No. It's a doll house. It just looks really real."

She paused, then decided.

"I think we should ask for it."

"Do you think that's okay?"

"We can ask."

She grabbed the catalogue and ran into the dining room where Mom and Dad were sitting at the table talking. They did that a lot.

"Look, Mommy. Isn't it beautiful?"

"Yes. It's a pretty price too," Mom answers.

"It's perfect. The most beautiful doll house ever made."

Dad is curious. "What have you found?"

"A doll house, Daddy. Look. It comes with furniture for every room, little toy people, a mom, a dad, and a baby. There's a swimming pool for the back, a driveway in the front, and a car. There's a lamp for the living room that works and the doorbell rings."

Dad takes the catalogue and looks over the glossy page.

"Well, that is pretty special, isn't it?"

"Yes! Do you think Santa could bring that for Christmas? I wouldn't care if I had nothing else."

Mom takes the catalogue from Dad.

"It's very expensive. I don't see how Santa can afford this."

"I wouldn't want anything else. Please."

Dad smiles down at Jayne and cups her hopeful face in his hands.

"Well, we'll see."

"Oh, thank you, Daddy! Thank you!" She throws her arms around his neck, and kisses his cheek, then runs back into the living room, beaming.

"Daddy said we'll see!"

Alone again in the dining room, Mom looks at Dad who is smiling at the picture of the most beautiful doll house ever made.

"Herb, how can you promise her that?"

"How can I not?"

Christmas morning our dad stood in the dining room doorway, coffee mug in hand, and smiled his crooked smile while his two little girls carefully set all the furniture in place in their beautiful, deluxe, very expensive doll house from the Simpson Sears catalogue.

It would be our last Christmas with our dad.

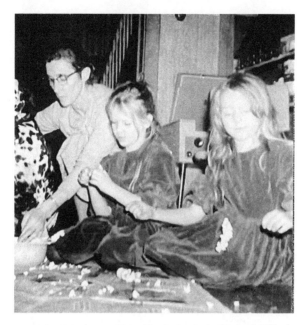

Christmas in our home on River Road (circa1962)
(Our dog, Caesar, Mom, Jayne, Winnifred)

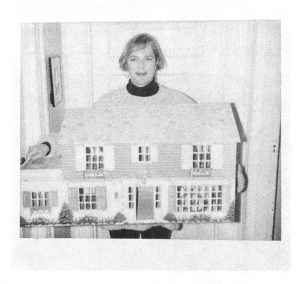

"I feel like only two men in my whole life have really loved me for who I am.
And they both bought me the same Doll House!"

*　　*　　*

The memory comes quickly and overwhelms her. She is a child again. It's that Christmas again.

Mother is packing. Cathy is worried. Father has assured her that Christmas holidays in the Highlands will be beautiful. Still, she cannot help but be concerned. When they asked her what she wanted Santa to bring her for Christmas she had no hesitation in asking for the doll house, and father had said that that was a wonderful thing to ask for. But they were leaving in a few days. They wouldn't be here on Christmas morning. How would Santa know where to deliver her gift?

"Well, why don't you write to Santa," Mother suggested, "And ask him to come a day early, before we leave?"

"Do you think he would?" Cathy was excited by that possibility.

Mother answered without looking up from her task of rolling socks and folding sweaters.

"I'm sure he would. Write him a letter and leave it here beside the fireplace. That way he's sure to find it."

That night before bed Cathy composes her letter.

Dear Santa,

I have tried to be a very good girl this year. I obey my parents and my teacher and I go to Church every Sunday. Mother says that I should write and tell you that we will not be at home this Christmas. Father is taking us to visit my Grandma and Grandpa in Kincardineshire. Mother says that I should tell you what I'd like for Christmas this year. I am very grateful for all the presents you gave me last year but this year I only want one thing and Father says it is a good gift to ask for. I would like a doll house, please. Would you please bring it a day early so I can take it with me to my Grandpa's house?

Thank you.

I hope you have a Happy Christmas.

Sincerely, Cathy Smith

Cathy folded the letter in half and the next morning before leaving for school she set it on the large hearth in front of their huge fireplace. Santa was sure to see it there tonight after she had gone to bed.

The school day seemed to drag on forever and when it finally ended Cathy rushed home. She would have supper and go to bed early to make the night come sooner.

"Catherine!" her mother met her at the door. "Have you been running?"

"No, Mother."

"I should hope not. It's very unseemly."

"Yes, Mother."

"By the way, Santa was here. He took your letter away."

Cathy could not believe her ears!

"He was here? In the daytime? You saw him?"

"Oh, yes." Mother was so matter of fact about it. "He came down the chimney and just picked up your letter."

"Did you talk to him? Did you tell him I was a good girl?"

"Yes, yes. I told him to come a day early this year, because we were going to be away, and he said he would."

"Oh, thank you, Mommy! Thank you!"

Cathy was beside herself with excitement. This would be the best Christmas ever.

It's December twenty-third, a cold, damp morning. She wakes and remembers that it's the day they leave. Mother has packed everything and set it by the door ready to go as soon as gifts have been opened and breakfast has been had. Cathy sits up in bed and waits for her mother to call her into the parlour. She can hardly contain herself, thinking of the how Santa has been to only her home to deliver the coveted doll house. No one else will be getting their gifts today. Only Cathy. Everyone else will have to wait until Christmas Eve. But not Cathy! It made her feel so special.

She can hear her parents' muffled voices and the clinking of teacups. She smells the fireplace burning, warming the parlour. It must be nearly time. And then her mother's voice sings out, "Cathy! Come see. Santa has been here!"

She flies out of the bed and runs to her door. Oh, no! Slippers. She swivels back around into the room and slides her feet into her slippers. Out the door. No. No. A robe. She must wear a robe. She grabs it from the foot of her bed and shoves her arms into the robe as she races now through the door and into the hallway. Her mother and father are standing in the doorway to the parlor, smiling. "Happy Christmas!" they say in unison.

"Happy Christmas, Mother! Happy Christmas, Father!" She hugs them each individually and then they step aside to let her into the room.

A bright fire burns in the fireplace. The parlor table is set with cups, saucers, and a steaming pot of tea. There are shortbread cookies arranged on a china plate and scones still hot from the oven smelling delicious. Hanging from the mantle is a singular stocking. A red and white striped stick of rock candy peeks out the top of the sock where a small sprig of holly is pinned. There is nothing else. Cathy stands and stares.

Her father places his hand on her shoulder.

"Well, go on, dear. Santa left that for you."

But Cathy does not move. She scans the room, searching for the promised gift but it's not here. Then her mother suggests,

"Take it down for her, Jim. It's much too high for her to reach."

"Of course! Here you are dear."

Her father hands Cathy the stocking.

"Open it up. Let's see what Santa gave you."

She sits on the settee beside the blazing fire and begins to empty the stocking. Rock candy. A colouring book. A ribbon for her hair. A small bag of chestnuts. Three pieces of ribbon candy and an orange.

"Isn't that nice!" her father exclaims. "I can't tell you how often I wished I had an orange when I was on the Continent. You know, they are very delicious and very good for you! Keeps the scurvy away!" he laughs.

"Oh, Jim. Stop it." her mother chides. "Well, dear Cathy. Happy Christmas."

The words stick in her throat, but the child manages, "Happy Christmas. Thank you, Mother. Thank you, Father."

"Don't thank us," her mother says. "Thank Santa! He knows what kind of little girl you are."

She wipes a tear away. He knows. Santa knows.

Herb is standing in the dining room doorway, coffee mug in hand, smiling his crooked smile while his girls play with their new doll house. "Look how happy they are, Cathy," he says. He was right, of course, to give it to them despite what she had said. He knows it may be their last Christmas together.

*　　*　　*

Jayne and I have been visiting Mr. and Mrs. Belzner, who are friends of our parents. Their son, Johnny, picked us up from home one afternoon and drove us to their farm near Port Colborne, only a half hour away. Just why we've been taken out of school for two weeks and sent to their farm no one explains. But it's a treat for us—an adventure. Belzner's farm has cows with long horns. That is where the warm milk comes from. We eat a jelly kind of thing called head cheese and brush our teeth with baking soda. Johnny Belzner is a young man and very kind to both of us.

"Come sit up on my lap and I'll read to you." Johnny says.

Jayne sits on one knee, and I sit on the other. Johnny gives us each a gentle hug. I hug him back. His whiskers rub my cheek.

"Just like Daddy." I say. "Jaynie, doesn't Johnny's beard feel just like Daddy's?"

He sort of smells like Daddy too. Tobacco.

"Yeah," my sister agrees. She notices a tear rolling down Johnny's cheek.

"What's the matter?" Jayne wants to know.

He lifts each of us off his lap and goes into the kitchen leaving us together by the chair. A moment later, Mrs. Belzner comes into the living room and sits us down on the couch—one on either side of her.

"Girls, I have something to tell you. Your daddy has gone to live with Jesus."

"What?"

"He's in heaven now. He's gone to live with Jesus."

Why would he do that, I wonder? But then, I think I understand what she's saying. Our dad has died. Died and gone to heaven. I look at my sister. She looks at me. We have no idea what to do with this news.

"You can cry if you want to. Go on. Put your head down here and cry."

So, I do. Is it because she told me to? I haven't really processed the news, but she said to cry. I cry.

My sister does not. Jayne sits quietly and shrugs off Mrs. Belzner's attempts to comfort her.

Soon after, we find ourselves back home again on River Road. Mom is wearing black—a new dress we've never seen before. The house is quiet, but the dining room table is covered in plates of food, like a church tea or a bridal shower.

Our dad is not here. We don't know how long he's been gone. The last time we saw him he was leaving by the kitchen door like so many times before, a small case in hand, a kiss goodbye and into Emerson Nix's car with Mom. Only Paul was home with Jayne and me as we watched our dad leave. Paul watched out the side bay window as the car left. He walked through the house, following the car as it rounded the corner of Almond Street and turned up River Road. He stood in the living room, watching it through the front window and stared as it rolled out of sight, as though willing it to return. And when it was well and truly gone our brother threw his body down onto the couch and sobbed into his arms.

"Don't cry, Paul," I said, softly patting his back. "It's okay. Daddy will be back. He always comes back."

But we never see him again. He died on February 4. It was a Monday.

* * *

I've never seen an apartment before much less one above a department store. The man with the keys leads Mom, Jayne, and I through the glass door on Main Street and up the stairs. There are two doors. He takes the keys and opens the one to the right.

"Right this way."

There's a smell that's vaguely familiar, like a place that has been closed up and longs for an open window. Where have I smelled that before?

"This is the living room. Two large south-facing windows overlooking Main Street. Of course, you'll have to provide your own curtains."

Mom stands in the middle of the dingy room, mentally arranging what furniture she could bring with her.

"And this is your kitchen. It's a galley kitchen. Fridge, stove, cupboards, sink."

It's not much more than a hallway between two rooms.

"Just this? Where would the table go?"

"If you want a table, you can put it in the room at the front of the apartment."

Mom is not impressed. For the price it should have a dining room or at least space for a table in the kitchen.

I am fascinated by the front of the sink. The wood panel there has several slits cut into it. Is it for decoration? What is it? Jayne isn't sure either.

"That's for ventilation. Please don't poke your fingers through there."

He must have read our minds.

The bedrooms are very small and there are only two. The window in one bedroom faces the brick wall of the building next door.

"Hmmm." Mom barely looks at the tiny rooms. "I don't know."

Jayne knows.

"There's no room for Paul."

"Who's Paul?"

80

"My son."

"A teenage son?"

"Yes. What has that to do with anything?"

"We couldn't tolerate unnecessary noise in this apartment, given that it's situated above a store."

"Paul doesn't make unnecessary noise." Jayne jumps to our brother's defence and is met with a stern look from Mom.

"Well, I'm not at all sure it's right for us. Not sure at all."

I walk back into the room at the front of the place. "Could we put the piano here?"

"Piano! No, Ma'am. You couldn't possibly have a piano in this apartment. As I've said, we can't tolerate unnecessary noise above the store during store hours. That includes loud play," he says, looking at Jayne and me, "and loud music. Even if you could get it up the stairs, you wouldn't be permitted to play it during store hours."

Not permitted to play it! Not permitted, by a store, to play my own piano?! It's not just *my* piano but I play it most. Daddy taught me to play "Cockles and Mussels" on it. He plays "Barbara Allen." Played. I mean, he *played* "Barbara Allen." Before. And when their friend Alfred Weiner visited, he said it was the most beautiful sounding piano he'd played since before the war.

We won't move here. I know it now. Mom would never leave our piano behind. Never. We've had that piano ever since we moved into the big house on River Road. That's where I smelled this before! When we first saw the house on River Road. It was empty too and smelled like this. Like it needed air. And love. But we won't be loving this place.

The man with the keys is opening the apartment door now and waiting for us to leave.

"You'll have to let me know by the end of the week if you think this will suit you."

"Thank you. Come on, girls."

Mom ushers us out the door and we run down the stairs, making unnecessary noise.

We're walking down Main Street now, headed to Merritt Park to sit for a while. Jayne takes my hand then looks up at Mom. "We're not going to live there, are we Mom?"

"No. We are not."

I knew Mom wouldn't leave my piano behind. As we cross the street in front of the bridge the siren sounds, signalling that the lift bridge is about to go up. A boat! Quickly now, to the park so that Jayne and I can run down the canal bank and stick our feet in the water. We sit on flat rocks splashing in the canal water until the ship goes by. It pulls the water away, smoothing the seaweed flat like silk and pulling small crabs and various creatures out of hiding. But the best part is once the ship has passed. Then the water rushes back in big waves that splash our feet and sometimes soak our clothes. It's the best part of being at Merritt Park.

Mom sits on a bench facing the canal. There wasn't much time left now. She'd have to find a place soon. But she was so unprepared for the search. How did this happen?

"How did this happen?" Kay thought. "When that piano came into our home, I never imagined we would ever have to move it. We would never have to move. It was a beautiful instrument. That woman! That community nurse! Imagine, coming to my hospital bed and telling me what a beautiful sounding piano we had. That meant she had been in the house when no one was there. The children were all staying with friends. That meant she had walked through our home, looked in our rooms, played our piano. Oh, my head. How did this happen?

I remember that I was walking to the grocery store. I stopped and spoke briefly with Frances Turnbull. She offered her condolences. Such a lovely man, she said. So sad for you and the children. Frances was sincere. She was always sincere. An artist with truth in her veins.

I was walking to the grocery store. Frances had got me thinking about Herb. That last night in the hospital. They called me to his bed. It's very soon now, they said. I held his hand. I prayed for his peace. I was thinking about Herb. He had been right about the mortgage. There hadn't been enough in the life insurance to cover it. I should have listened to him.

I should have . . .

I was walking to the grocery store. The ringing in my ears grew loud. My whole body was shaking. I felt . . . I think I'm going to . . . cement. I'm on the cement sidewalk in front of the grocery store. Someone is calling my name. Herb? Is that you?"

"Just take it easy, Mrs. Bray. There's an ambulance on the way."

Where did they take me? One hospital. And then another. Dr. White must have been called. I don't remember. After those treatments, those shock treatments, there was so much I couldn't remember. "Please don't cry, Mrs. Bray. Try to calm down," they said. "It's all right. It's all right," they said.

But it wasn't all right. It was hell.

It's not all right! My head. Don't touch my head. Don't. Don't ride your bike. You need to keep your red cells up . . . right up there by the roof. There's water coming in! Daddy! We're going to sink! We're going to sink . . . at the grocery store . . . not all right."

*   *   *

In the end, Mom found an apartment without our assistance or opinion. But I suspect that she may have had some help from our big brother.

Jim worked with Stubby Wilkes down at the Welland Flour and Feed, and Stubby's mother owned an apartment building.

It was a square, four-unit building on Frazer Street and looked like a large Lego block covered in artificial brick. There was no front porch. No trees. No screen door. Just two sets of wooden stairs, one in front of the other, that ran up the outside of the building.

The cement walk between the apartment building and the I.O.O.F. Meeting Hall next door ended at the entrance to one of the ground floor flats. Three steps up from the sidewalk in front was the door to another flat and our new home was on top of that. Affixed to the small landing at the top of the wobbly stairs was a wooden pole for the clothesline that ran to the back of the building.

Everything had been moved in by the time Jayne and I saw the place. Fait accompli. A done deal.

The old wooden door opened into a square room with no window. And no furniture. Only another door on the other side.

"What's this?" I asked.

"Well, it's the first room. Like an entry," Mom explained. "I think it will be our dining room."

"Where's the table?

"I couldn't bring the dining room suite. I gave it to Betty and Jim . . . as a wedding gift."

So, the family dining room table, six chairs, buffet, and china cabinet did not make the move. How would this ever be a dining room, we wondered?

Through the door at the far end of the room we found ourselves facing a long hallway to the left, a kitchen to the right, and what was obviously the bathroom in front of us. It had a cast-iron claw-foot tub like the one at home—our old home—a small, mirrored cabinet above the sink, a toilet, of course, and an odd-looking metal tank next to the window.

"What's that?" I asked again.

"That is the water heater. You must never touch it. Only Paul or I will light it."

"Light it?"

"Yes," Mom answered me. "This cylinder on the side opens so that you can light it and heat the water in the tank. Look. See the coils? The water runs through those and is heated. But once the tank is hot you must turn it off or else it will explode. So, you must never touch it. Do you understand?"

Jayne, who had said nothing so far, frowned..

"So there's no hot water."

"Of course there's hot water. Just not all the time. You have to turn on the tank."

"Oh brother." And Jayne left the bathroom.

We met her in the large kitchen around the corner. This room had its own door too. In fact, it had two doors. The second, we were to learn in the time to come, led to the apartment behind us. It was locked with a hook and an eye latch.

Down the long hallway, we passed a little alcove and another door to a cubby hole. This would be the perfect spot for the piano, I thought. We passed a bedroom with a large wooden wardrobe for a closet, our parents' highboy, and one of our brothers' bunk beds. This was Paul's room.

At the front of the apartment was the living room. Sitting as it did on the corner of the building it had two large windows. One in front and one on the side. From the side window, you could see down Frazer Street to the Welland Flour and Feed where Jim worked. In the corner of the living room was a big square heater. A metal pipe snaked from the behind the thing and ran straight up to the top of the tall ceiling. This was meant to heat the entire apartment. Next to the heater was one more door which Jayne opened.

"What's this?"

"Our bedroom," Mom replied.

There was our parents' bed and dresser and another free-standing wardrobe that was the closet.

"Where's our room?" I heard a bit of panic in my sister's voice.

"There are only two bedrooms. You girls will share with me."

Jayne and I looked at each other. Where was our four-poster bed?

"But there's no room in here for our bed," my sister dared.

"No. I gave it away."

She gave it away? Gave it away?

"But it's our bed!" I protested.

"There was no room for it. You girls will be fine with me."

Now I noticed that Dad's La-Z-Boy chair wasn't here either. No dining room suite. No La-Z-Boy. No four-poster bed. I was almost afraid to ask, but I did.

"And the piano?"

"I was told it wouldn't make it up the stairs."

Gone. Like every trace of our lives on River Road, it was gone.

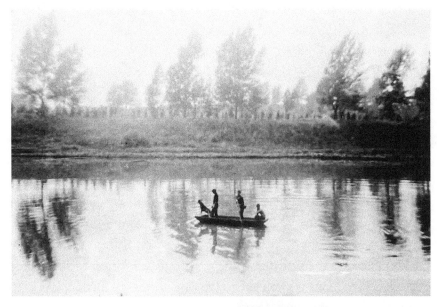

Paul captaining his first boat on the Welland River
with our dog, Caesar, and two friends.

PART TWO

TITHING

It was nearly September and time to go back to school. But not Riverview School because now we lived on the other side of the canal.

It was all new to us, this other side of Welland. New home, neighbours, and stores. And a different school with different classmates and teachers. The only true consolation for Jayne and I was the fact that we would be in the same class, Jayne having been held back once more. We would both be in Grade Four together.

A few days before classes began, Mom walked us over to the school so we could learn the route and have a look at Queen Street School. We walked up Frazer Street away from our flat and crossed West Main. We passed the Four Square Gospel Church on the corner. That was when the neighbourhood changed. There were no apartment buildings or meeting halls here. No bank or Welland Hotel. There were tall trees that shaded the sidewalk and houses that boasted porches and gardens. We passed two stately homes, situated side by side, each on a different corner of the same street. Both houses were large but very different from each other. One looked to me like a Southern mansion. It was a two-storey white house with a flat roof and wide veranda that ran all across the front and around one side of the house. On the corner, the veranda jutted out into the yard to form a huge circular sitting area. The roof of the veranda was held up by no less than twelve pillars. To me it seemed regal and I immediately fell in love with this house.

"Oh, I would love to live there!" I said, stopping to admire my fantasy home.

But Jayne said, "Not me." as she stood looking at the house next door. "This one is mine."

I had, in my imagination, claimed the first beautiful house we saw because it was big and white and elegant looking. But Jayne was drawn to the pseudo-Tudor house next door. Not that we knew what a Tudor house was back then. Still, Jayne's tastes clearly ran to the more refined and quietly gracious. Her choice of home was also set back from the street and had a wide, deep front yard. The lawn was shaded by tall trees on either side. Seven wide steps up from the long front walk was a generous veranda that also wrapped around the house. But its peaked roof was firmly supported by dependable, square posts. Between the posts ran a railing of dark wood with white spindles where gentle breezes could waft across its visitors while at the same time promising quiet privacy. This entry seemed warmer in its welcoming than the openness of the house I had claimed. Every window had its own character in size and shape. Unique. On the second floor was a small, private balcony where Jayne clearly imagined herself sipping tea. Every aspect of the house spoke to Jayne.

"This is where I want to live." She said with a decisiveness that was more a statement than a wish.

"That is a family estate," Mom said, when she turned to see that her girls were no longer following her. "You could never afford to live there even if it were someday for sale. Come on now, girls. This way."

And with that Mom broke us from our fanciful reverie. We followed her further up the street and around the corner where Queen Street School soon loomed before us, a large, two and a half-storey brick and stone building. Jayne stopped dead in her tracks.

"It looks like Central School." she said, apprehension in her voice.

Central School where she had been held back a year and the teacher was nuts.

"Yes, well, they were built at about the same time," Mom answered. "But this one is newer."

Newer! It did not look "newer" to us. Riverview School was newer, nicer, and closer to home. It didn't have a second floor like this building. Jayne was right. This building looked like Central School except maybe a little smaller. The windows were different too. There was a covered stone stairway that led up to the front double doors, but we did not go up the stairs. Mom took us around to the side of the building and a second set of doors.

"This is where you girls will go in." she said. "I'll come in with you on the first day just to make sure you know where to go. All right?"

"All right," Jayne answered. I nodded.

"You'll be fine. You're going to make all kinds of new friends, and you'll be together the whole time."

I took hold of Jayne's hand.

"Okay." My sister conceded, sounding not quite convinced.

All too soon summer ended. Labour Day came and went and before we knew it, we were on our way to the first day of Grade Four.

The school yard was full of kids of all ages. Some girls playing skip rope, some boys playing tag. There was laughter and yelling, calling out of names, and a general air of excitement as friends greeted each other for the first day of school. There were also two new faces, a major curiosity that drew whispers and giggles as Jayne and I followed Mom through the throng.

We walked through the side doors of the school, up the stairs, and through a second set of doors. There was a wide hallway with gleaming wooden floors and several closed classroom doors. Our anxious, thumping hearts echoed in our ears and bounced off the high ceiling.

"This way," Mom said as she led us down the hall and stopped in front of the principal's office. That's what the sign on the door read. Principal's Office. She knocked and a kind face opened the door.

"Mrs. Bray," he said. "I'm Vice-Principal Farnsworth. We're expecting you and your girls. Please come in."

"Thank you." Mom replied as she walked into the office. Jayne and I followed.

Mr. Farnsworth smiled as he stepped behind the desk.

"Please sit down, Mrs. Bray," he offered, and Mom took the only other chair. "Principal Huck is delayed at present, so he has asked me to make sure you are properly enrolled this morning. I understand you know him from his previous posting."

"Yes," Mom replied. "Melvin Huck was principal at Riverview School when our girls attended there. My husband and I knew him quite well."

He read something on the desk and then looked up at us saying, "So, this must be Jayne and Winnifred."

"Yes," Mom answered.

"Well, welcome girls," he said directly to us. "I hope you will settle into Queen Street School easily." Then reading again, "And you are both in Grade Four. Twins?"

Jayne groaned, quietly.

"Not twins." Mom answered. "They are fifteen months apart. Jayne is the eldest."

"I see. Well, we'll just sign a few things here, Mrs. Bray, and we can take the girls to class once the bell rings." Then he spoke directly to Jayne and to me again. "Your teacher's name is Mrs. Gorbet. She's expecting you."

Soon after, the school bell rang and the sound of excited young voices and scampering footsteps echoed outside the principal's office. We waited. When the halls grew quiet again Mr. Farnsworth led Mom, Jayne, and me to our new classroom where he gently knocked on the closed door. One moment later it opened, and there stood our new teacher, Mrs. Gorbet She smiled and said, "Hello." Just as though we were neighbours stopping by for tea.

"Good morning, Mrs. Gorbet," Mr. Farnsworth replied. "This is Mrs. Bray and her two daughters, Jayne and Winnifred, who have come to join your class."

"Hello, Mrs. Bray. Nice to meet you." And she shook Mom's hand.

"Thank you. Nice to meet you, too." Mom replied. "I'll leave you girls now and see you at home for lunch." Then she kissed each of us on the top of our head and left.

"I've been expecting you, Jayne, Winnifred. Come in. We are all just getting to know each other." She opened the door wider, stepped through it, and turned to invite us in. Then she stood between us and placed her hands on our each of our shoulders while she spoke to the class.

"We have two new students at Queen Street School this year. This is Jayne and Winnifred Bray and I'm happy to say that they will be your classmates this year. I know that you will make them feel welcome."

A few heads nodded amiably while a few more faces stared at the curiosity of new kids in the room.

"Jayne,' Mrs. Gorbet said. "I have a desk for you right here. And one for you, Winnifred just a couple rows away. Have a seat." She smiled. So we did. Then she spoke to the class.

"I'm very glad to have all of you in my classroom for grade four. Some of you are already friends from last year. And some of you have not yet met. So, we're going to spend some time this morning getting acquainted by talking about your summer. And then we'll take time so that you can write your memories down. Is there anyone who would like to tell us what they've been doing during summer vacation?"

A few hands went up. But I didn't really listen to what was being said. I was still hearing Mrs. Gorbet's voice in my head. It was so lovely to listen to. There was no stern disciplined air about her like my grade-one teacher. No tiresome sighs like my teacher in grade two. Mrs. Gorbet was kind and calm. And she made me calm in return. I looked over at Jayne who must have sensed my smile because she turned her head and smiled back at me. Maybe it would be all right after all.

It was quiet time now. We had all been given paper and pencil and time to write our stories down. I hadn't shared anything out loud with the class. Neither had Jayne. But I would think of something that only Mrs. Gorbet would read because I trusted that she would keep it to herself, especially if I asked her to. She just seemed like a trustworthy teacher. The classroom was quiet except for the scratching of pencils and the occasional sniff or cough. Mrs. Gorbet sat at her desk watching us work and getting up from time to time to discreetly help someone with spelling or remembering. I saw her pass by Jayne, look down at her work and gently touch the top of my sister's head. I wondered what she was reading.

Suddenly there was a knock at the door. Mrs. Gorbet answered it, quietly spoke to whoever was there, and then stepped out into the hallway. Everyone stopped working. The teacher had left the room! We heard muffled voices that seemed to rise and fall like a quiet argument. And then silence.

In the next moment, Mrs. Gorbet came back into the classroom followed by Vice-Principal Farnsworth and a tall, slim, grey-haired man, Principal Huck. A charge of anxiousness ran through the classroom. What did the principal want? Who were they here for? We all held our breath.

Then, Mrs. Gorbet walked over to Jayne, knelt beside her desk, and said softly, "I'm sorry, dear, but it seems you've been placed in the wrong class."

"What do you mean?" Jayne asked.

"This isn't your class, dear. We need to move you."

"No. We're to stay together." Jayne protested, pointing at me.

"There's been a mistake and we need to take you to another class."

The look that Jayne threw me at that moment sent a shock of fear through me. But she did not move from her desk. No one moved.

The silence in the classroom amplified every word that was being spoken. Everyone was listening.

Principal Huck stepped further into the room.

"Thank you, Mrs. Gorbet. We'll take care of this." He looked directly at Jayne and said, "Come with us now. Mr. Farnsworth will get you sorted out."

Mrs. Gorbet reluctantly stood, never taking her eyes from Jayne who got up, slowly picking up her paper and pencil.

"Leave that. You won't need it," Principal Huck said.

Jayne walked past him and looked back at me, two rows over. Helpless. We were helpless.

Then Principal Huck said, "Upstairs to the Grade Three room, Mr. Farnsworth."

The room gasped.

"Thank you, Mrs. Gorbet. You can resume your lesson now."

Jayne stopped and dropped her head. But he gave her a little nudge and my sister disappeared out the door without another look back at the humiliation left in the room.

*   *   *

Camp Maple Leaf was the best camp in the world! Not that we had anything to compare it to . . . yet. Two weeks on an island somewhere north of Peterborough. Maybe it was one week. I don't actually recall how long we were there. I only know it was the best summer of our lives so far. The camp was on an island, so you had to take a boat to get there. Well, really it was a barge. There was a long dock, a large clubhouse where we had great meals, and a canteen where you could buy snacks. And there were several cabins housing six girls each plus a counsellor. Boys came to camp on different weeks. The canteen was great because the counsellors gave you each a dime every day that you could spend right away or save up for something really good like a giant chocolate bar.

Jayne and I weren't in the same cabin because she was older. Fifteen months, but that was enough to place her with the seniors. I didn't mind. All the counsellors had nicknames like Skippy or Angel. Twinkle was our counsellor. I remember her as tiny, like Tinker Bell, but not as feisty.

There was a mini-Olympics day, a talent contest, canoe lessons and an outdoor sleepover somewhere at the other end of the island. The older girls took canoes to their private campsite while my age group was transported in the barge. We had a campfire and roasted marshmallows, but no one told spooky stories or anything like that. We mostly just talked and got to know each other. I remember sleeping under large tarps stretched between trees. Not the most comfortable sleep given the hard roots we bunked down on. But I didn't mind.

I didn't see a lot of Jayne except at meals, which were great! And then she sat with the girls from her cabin, as we all did.

My first mistake at camp was when I ran in the mini-Olympics. I was chosen as one of the runners from our cabin in the relay race. I would be the last runner. When we were all in place Counsellor Twinkle came up to our group and pointed to the white post on the other side of a small grove of trees. That was where we were supposed to run to. Got it. I surveyed the route I would take. Over this ditch, around that big tree and then straight on to the post. I even told the girl next to me that that was my plan. I thought it was a pretty good one. Cap gun bang! Cheers! Go! Go! Go! I was ready. Suddenly I was tagged on the shoulder and off I went. Over the ditch, around that big tree, and then straight on to the post. I won! The counsellor at the white post didn't see me come in, but when she turned around, there I was. First place.

Then the girl who had stood next to me arrived. "She cheated!"

"What?"

What was she talking about? I had won.

"She cheated. She ran through the woods."

The counsellor looked at me.

"Did you? Which way did you come?"

"Straight across there."

"You left the road?"

"What road?"

"You were supposed to stay on the road and run around the trees."

"Oh."

Someone should have told us that. But I guess I was the only one who wasn't familiar with the rules of relay. One thing I was familiar with was embarrassment. Even here at Camp Maple Leaf. And that I did mind.

At the time, we didn't know that Camp Maple Leaf was for needy children. I don't remember feeling needy most of time. Although I'm sure we looked it to much of the world. To feel needy, I suppose you would have to compare yourself to others around you. It was enough for a ten-year-old to just be. Naïve, unaware? Perhaps. Not oblivious, though, to the comments of store clerks, teachers, or parents of possible friends who found you lacking in some way.

"Mom, this is my friend from school," Amy tells her mother. "We're going over to the swings at Chippewa Park."

One quick assessment was all it took.

"Not today," my new friend's mother replies.

"But why? I don't have any homework."

"You're not a very clean little girl to be going anywhere, are you?"

"But we're going to play on the swings. I'll get dirty anyway."

"A young girl should always be clean. Say goodbye to your friend and come downstairs."

That was the one and only time I was ever in Amy's house. It was a big white wooden home on a street right across from the canal. Upstairs she had her very own bedroom with a canopy bed that was fully and neatly made up in ruffled pink and white and a dresser with her very own mirror. And she kept her sweaters in a drawer. None of this seemed unusual to her. I suppose because, to her, it wasn't unusual. And I don't remember Amy ever calling me friend again. She never explained why. I just seemed to disappear from her world.

It was like that. I never really noticed the difference between kids my own age and me. Not at ten years old, anyway. But their parents were often more discerning. Perhaps, discriminating is a better word. Still, you don't always need words to dish out shame on a child.

The following year, Camp Maple Leaf only had room for one of us. And since it was the last year that Jayne would be young enough to attend it was decided that she should go. I would instead go to the Salvation Army Summer Camp, somewhere near Lake Simcoe. Camp Maple Leaf it was not.

The Salvation Army Summer Camp was touted as "A place where underprivileged youths could get away from their everyday surroundings and enjoy nature." I remember getting away. I don't recall much nature. The camp's aim was to 'meet health, spiritual education, social and recreational need through creative, safe and fun experiences.' I don't know that I had many spiritual needs. More and more I seemed to spend a lot of time in church with Mom as Jayne spent less and less.

Like Maple Leaf, this camp had cabins with six campers each. Every morning we were required to make our bunks before inspection. Tight sheets and mitered corners were required of every bed if our cabin was to win the daily award for neatness. So, each day we struggled to spread and tuck and tighten our bedding. The top bunks were the most difficult to bring up to code given that our cabin was mostly made up of very short people. But try as we may, we never passed inspection. And so, the daily award of the Niagara Falls snow globe never graced our breakfast table. You only got to keep the award for the day, but breakfast bragging rights was something to be coveted, nonetheless.

Boys and girls attended camp at the same time. That was different from Maple Leaf too. The camp was made up of two long lines of cabins separated by a large playing field. Boys on one side. Girls on the other. Every morning, after inspection and before breakfast, we were required to stand outside facing the cabins on the other side. And every morning a small group of campers invariably walked the length of that field carrying their wet bedding in a humiliating march to the laundry house for all to see. Something about that seemed less Salvation and more Army to me and I don't believe it bolstered anyone's spiritual education.

Breakfast was porridge, toast, and milk which suited me just fine. Of course, there was Grace followed by the Lord's Prayer before every meal, and if you didn't know the words to the Lord's Prayer when you arrived at camp you certainly knew them by the time you left. Chapel was visited at least once a day.

After breakfast, the head counsellor outlined the day's activities. Craft time, sports time, nap time, next meal, and so on. Sports time was usually a soccer game for the boys on the large field. Craft time turned out to be pasting burned wooden matches to cardboard in the shape of a crucifix. From the activity room, you could see the large cement swimming pool where the sunlight glistened on the blue chlorinated water. Every morning I said my own silent prayer that today we would go swimming. Every morning my prayers were not answered. That is, not until the last day of camp when an afternoon of swimming was announced as a kind of reward for being such good, Christian campers.

*   *   *

Frank and Charlotte Gorbet had a lovely home on Church Street, just a ten-minute walk from our apartment. Once a month Mom took the ten dollars saved from her Family Allowance cheque and walked to Gorbet's to give them the cash. She was tithing.

The first time she did this they were pleased to see her even though the visit was unexpected. Mom just rang their bell and was welcomed into their home for tea. Then she handed Charlotte the little brown pay envelope and said, "I want to contribute to the State of Israel cause. Would you please see that this money is sent to the proper place?"

"How very kind of you, Kay," Frank responded, rather surprised by the gesture. "But are you sure you want to do this?"

"Absolutely." There was no doubt in her mind. The Children of Israel had come home as foretold in Scripture which meant that these were surely the Final Days before the Rapture. Anything she could do to help bring that about she would do.

Frank and Charlotte thanked her for her thoughtful gift and accepted what they assumed to be a onetime offering. But it was not. Every month for many months, Kay Bray arrived at their home and handed over the envelope for The Cause. Eventually they convinced her that the State of Israel appreciated her contribution but no longer needed her ten dollars. Mom reluctantly agreed. So, the money began to go, instead, to the Four Square Gospel Church.

One day, over tea and Mandelbrot cookies, Charlotte said to her, "Kay, you are such an intelligent woman. Can't you see that your Church doesn't need that money? *You* do. Your girls are growing up. They'll be teenagers soon and they'll start dating. You need to get a telephone for those girls."

A telephone. Yes, she supposed a telephone would be useful for a lot of things. Perhaps Charlotte was right.

The next month the phone arrived and was installed in the hallway just outside of Paul's bedroom door. It sat on the recently acquired telephone table, complete with a brown and orange upholstered seat on one side and a space below for the telephone book. It was a small, added expense, but somehow there was still enough money every month for tithing to the Four Square Gospel Church.

*　　*　　*

"The Lord is my shepherd. I shall not want. He maketh me to lie down in green pastures. He leadeth me beside the still waters . . ."[1]

I know this one. It's easy to remember because I've heard it over and over again. At every church or fellowship gathering we've ever attended, be it inside, outside, under open sky or in a canvas tent, there will almost assuredly be a reciting of the twenty-third Psalm. So I know this one. And I'm certain that I'm going to win the prize for memorizing it.

But the church lady standing in front of me doesn't seem convinced. In fact, she seems quite provoked that I, a ragged ten-year-old with long, unruly hair, should presume to win anything at all. And anyway, what would I do with a lovely piece of fine china bric-a-brac crafted into a tiny bouquet of roses and donated to the Sunday School by the church lady herself as a generous Christian gesture. Who was I to presume? Still, here I was.

Sunday School has finished and Sister Ketchum, the Pastor who lives with her family in the cold two-bedroom basement apartment of this Four Square Gospel Church, is beginning Sunday service in the sanctuary. I've already been attended to once by some other church lady who sympathized that my mother obviously didn't own a hairbrush, but wasn't it lovely to see a child making an effort to attend Sunday service all on her own. She's tied my hair back with a rag of her own hanky torn in half.

"Yea, though I walk through the valley of the shadow of death, I shall fear no evil."

I had thought that I'd get to go into the Pastor's office to recite. I'd seen others do it. I knew every part of this little church.

From the entry vestibule, richly panelled in dark, shiny wood, to the winding back stairs that led past the baptismal tank and through to the open lower floor Sunday School area right to the cold two-bedroom basement apartment where Mom and I sometimes visited

---

1. Psalm 23 - The Lord is my Shepherd – A Song of David - King James Bible

Sister Ketchum for tea. But I had never been inside the Pastor's office. Its gleaming, wooden door and brass doorknob now faced me, here in the vestibule, like a challenge to my faith. I could venture almost anywhere in this little church but entry to that room was off limits, it seemed.

"Surely goodness and mercy shall follow me all the days of my life and I shall dwell in the house of the Lord forever."

There. I've done it. The church lady looks at me and flatly says, "That's not right."

"What?" In my head I hear Mom correct me. "*Say Pardon.*"

"You haven't got it right," the church lady says.

"What did I get wrong?"

"I can't tell you that. Try it again if you want," sighs the guardian of the prize. Clearly, she doesn't think I know what I'm reciting.

But I do. This time I take my time and am very careful about each line. "Thou preparest a table before me in the presence of mine enemies." I've always liked that line about preparing a table. I'd imagined a banquet with platters of fruit, bread, and steaming meat. I'd never thought about the enemies part.

Now one of the double doors to the sanctuary opens and another church lady tiptoes out, softly closing the door behind her.

"What's going on?" she whispers.

"Oh, nothing," the first lady says. "She's trying to recite the twenty-third Psalm, but she can't get it right."

She's wrong. I know she is. But in my head, I hear Mom warn me, "*Respect your elders.*" So, I say nothing.

"Do you want to try again?" the kinder lady asks me.

"There's no point in that," snaps the generous, Christian donor of the gift. "What would she do with this prize anyway?" she decides aloud as she shows the fragile ornament.

"Oh, yes," admires the quiet Christian. Then she turns to me. "This is a very expensive piece meant for an older person, dear. Someone who can appreciate it. Why would a little girl like you want this? Perhaps when you are older, dear."

That seems to have decided it. The generous Christian turns away, opens the gleaming door, and steps through to the Pastor's office, taking the delicate prize and the meek Christian lady with her. They close the door behind them. I go home.

"What is in your hair?"

I'd forgotten about the rag, but Mom notices it almost as soon as she walks in the door. And she is not happy about it.

"Where did you get that?"

"One of the ladies at church tied my hair back."

"With a torn hanky!? Why?"

"I don't know. One lady said she didn't have a comb and so another lady said she would just tie it back for me."

"With a rag? What must they think of me? Oh. I'll never be able to show my face there again."

She covers her embarrassed face with both hands and plops down onto a kitchen chair.

"Sorry." It's all I can think to say. If only I had won the china ornament. She would have liked that.

The phone rings and as Mom gets up to answer it, she tells me to put the kettle on. I do. It's another church lady on the phone but from a different church. This is the skinny lady with the clenched hair who attends services with us in another church lady's house in Port Colborne. We usually go there whenever we can get a ride, and we stay all day because that's how long it takes for everyone to have their turn at preaching. The skinny lady with the clenched hair doesn't preach, but she loves to listen when Mom does. Mom thinks she is a very good and helpful friend. So it must be an answer to prayer that skinny church lady has called just when Mom needs her most.

I listen to Mom relate the hair rag story. She's humiliated. She's angry. She's ashamed that she is guilty of the sin of pride. But what can she do?

The kettle whistles and I make the tea.

Now I hear the familiar sound of muffled praise and pleas mixed with the sniffs of thankfulness. They're praying together. And it seems the prayers are about to be answered. What's required, I soon learn, is a way to keep my hair and my sister's hair tidy with very little maintenance. A perm is the very thing! We will not only be given professional hair perms in a real salon, but this church lady will make a gift of it. It will be part of her tithes. It will have to be at her salon in Port Colborne, though. Are we able to get a ride? Yes. Our big brother, Jim, will take us.

The following Saturday, my sister and I are in the salon, sitting side by side, each in our own chair and smiling into the large mirror at each other. Our adventure begins with the pump, pump, pump of our chairs being raised. We giggle. They tie an apron around each of us and now someone is lifting and handling my hair. It tickles and feels nice. It's the man who owns the salon and now he's trying to comb the knots out of my long waves. I've been through this before. It takes time, but it's achievable. Perhaps he doesn't have the time, though, because he says to the young woman getting ready to do Jayne's hair,

"You'd better use this conditioner or you're going to have the same mess I have here."

The skinny church lady with the clenched hair is standing behind Jayne. I don't know where Mom is, but she's not in the salon.

Suddenly church lady says, "Never mind that. Just cut it all off."

What did she say? Jayne speaks up.

"No! You can't cut my hair."

But through thin, grimacing lips the skinny church lady says, "Oh, yes I can."

The salon owner drops my hair and turns to her.

"Lady, I don't think I can do that. Are these your girls?"

"No, but their mother knows that they are here with me." She crosses her arms with authority.

"For a perm!" Jayne shouts. "You are supposed to perm our hair."

"Oh, Honey, your hair is much too fine to take a perm." says the sweet, soft spoken young woman combing out Jayne's hair.

But skinny church lady persists.

"I am telling you to cut it. Cut it all off. It's just a rat's nest."

"Lady, I can't be responsible for doing that. You're not their mother."

"I'll be responsible. I am paying for this, and I insist that you do as I say."

Now Jayne is screaming. "You can't cut our hair! Pooh Bray, they're trying to cut our hair!"

She does not make it easy for them. My big sister, who was always braver and more independently minded than I, wraps her arms around her head and continues yelling.

But in the end, she loses the battle. Sobbing, my sister closes her eyes so that she cannot see the long strands that fall into her lap and onto the floor. I've never seen Jayne in such defeat. I begin to cry too.

My hair was always thicker than Jayne's. Hers was fine and baby soft. It never tangled the way mine did. So, I cannot explain why mine was cut to shoulder length, but Jayne's was cropped up to her ears.

"It's a page boy," the young woman says softly to my sister. "Look how pretty you are."

"I hate it. I look like a boy." It's all she says.

The skinny, clenched church lady is putting her wallet away now. But she soon discovers that she has only begun to pay for her crime.

Standing in front of the salon we see our brother's car pull up. Mom is in the front seat with Jim. Jayne and I open the back door and climb in, still sobbing, as skinny Clench the Wench gets in the front seat next to Mom. Then, our brother turns to see why we're crying, and his face turns beat red. His temper explodes.

"What the hell? What the hell have you done to their hair!?"

The protests from skinny clenched lady, and the attempts to calm things by our mother are all drowned out by the barrage of our brother's fury.

"Who the hell do you think you are? You had no right to cut their hair! If you were a man, I'd punch you right in face. I don't care who she is. She had no right to cut their hair. Let her cry! She should cry. Look what you've done to her. I don't give a shit if she paid for it or not. She had no right. Don't tell me not to swear. It's my car! I'll say what I want."

I don't remember Mom saying anything more. I don't remember the rest of the ride home or dropping off the clenched church lady. I do remember that she was not as confident and bossy in my brother's car as she had been in the salon. Jim had effectively blasted the arrogance right out of her. But the damage of her sneaky deed had been done.

Jayne's hair never grew back to the length we both once had.

* * *

Union Carbide was hiring, and at eighteen, Paul was old enough to apply. It was one of the more desirable factories in Welland at which to be employed. Good, steady, clean work. Chemical work. Not hot steel factory work. Not a low-paying cotton mill job where so many high school dropouts ended up. Men who got into Union Carbide stayed there for years and retired with a steady pension. It was a good job, and it was just what Paul needed. He would quit his dishwashing job at the Chinese restaurant and start making real money. Mom would be able to quit her part time job at the *Evening Tribune*. And what a great Christmas they would have if he were bringing home a Union Carbide pay cheque. Early Monday morning Paul walked to the factory's main office and joined the line of hopefuls ready for steady work.

The application form was straightforward enough. Age, name, address, work experience. The next step was the physical—standard practice. Height, weight, blood pressure, and so on. After this he would join the hopeful men who occupied the room of chairs as they waited for their names to be called. But he never made it to that room. As he started to go, the doctor called him back.

"Paul Bray?" he said.

"Yes." Paul turned back.

"I'm sorry, but your application has been rejected."

"What? Why?"

"I am afraid that you've failed the physical. All plant employees must weigh at least one hundred thirty-five pounds. You are underweight by three pounds."

"Three pounds?"

"Afraid so. You should weigh at least a hundred and thirty-five. Especially at your height and age. Sorry. Thank you for applying to Union Carbide."

The doctor put his file aside and moved on.

Paul walked home slowly. His buddies always called him Ghost, a nickname born of his pale complexion. Today he felt like a ghost. Feather light and fading.

*   *   *

There were three variety stores in the neighbourhood. Lansky's, Kiraly's and the store of the skinny old man in the house next to the river. All three stores were created in what were formerly the front rooms of old houses.

Lansky's and Kiraly's were both on Main Street, side by side as a matter of fact. Mr. Lansky didn't like the Kiraly's because they didn't speak English very well and sold individual cigarettes to anyone with a dime, regardless of their age. Mr. and Mrs. Kiraly hated Mr. Lansky mostly because he was there, right next to their store, on purpose. At least, those were the reasons we thought they hated each other. But it could have been because one was a Lansky, the other a Kiraly.

As kids we preferred Mr. Lansky. He always understood what we said and always smiled. Because he lived in the back of the house you could often get a whiff of his dinner simmering on some unseen stove. But best of all he had a great penny candy counter and was never impatient as we thought and rethought how best to spend a nickel. Into the little brown paper bag Mr. Lansky would carefully drop the three-for-a-penny sweet tarts, two-for-a-penny coke bottle candies, a full penny liquorish pipe and two caramels. No! Wait. Instead of the coke bottle candies, a packet of Lick-a-Made. Cherry. Sweet tarts, liquorish pipe, caramels, and Lick-a-Made.

"No coke bottles?"

"Oh, yeah. I like those."

"What about two-for-a-penny coke bottle candies and one caramel instead of two?"

"Okay. Thanks."

Sometimes the second caramel would magically appear in the bag after all. So even though Kiraly's store was there first, Lansky's was the best place for a kid.

The store of the skinny old man in the house next to the river must have had a name but I don't remember what it was. It wasn't there for very long. It didn't have a candy counter or ten-cent cigarettes. It was more of a general store, really. Bare wooden floors, shelves stocked with canned goods of questionable age and a long counter behind which stood the skinny old man. At one end of his counter was a big white weigh scale where he would measure out dry goods. Flour, rolled oats, coffee beans, and sugar. One pound of sugar poured into a little brown paper bag and tied with white string could be had for ten cents. So his store was a kind of combination experience. Lansky's paper bag filled with sweetness for the price of Kiraly's single cigarette.

You couldn't help but wonder about the skinny old man. He was the only person you ever saw in the store, standing behind his counter but never leaning on it. And even though he never took his eyes off you while you were in his store you couldn't really see the colour of his eyes, so deeply set into his sad face were they. If he had had one leg, you might have thought him a veteran of the Great War. From time to time, you would see old men like that on Main Street walking with crutches, one pant leg pinned up to their thigh leaving a space where their other leg should be. But the skinny old man in the store next to the river had both legs. So, if he had left anything of himself on a battlefield in Europe it did not show from the outside.

Mom was thrilled to learn that I had discovered a store where sugar could be bought for ten cents a pound. Every week I was sent to the store next to the river with one thin dime specifically for that purpose. I don't know what the skinny old man thought about this rag-a-muffin kid who only ever bought sugar once a week. I didn't really care. I was so proud of my discovery, as though I was responsible for maintaining the family budget while providing Mom with her ever-essential sugar. With each purchase I became bolder, more confident in my request.

"One pound of white sugar, please." I would pronounce, placing the dime on the long counter.

It's possible that the skinny old man eventually decided his price for that condiment was far too low. It's possible, but I don't know. Because the day we didn't have a dime was the last day I ever went into his store.

"Just go and ask him if you can have the sugar and pay him tomorrow."

"He won't do that, Mom."

"It's only for one day, until I get my cheque."

"But we can have tea without sugar for one day."

"Oh, I can't bear that. I'd rather go hungry than drink tea without sugar."

I knew we wouldn't go hungry. There was a pot of barley soup on the stove and four cracked eggs in the fridge.

"You ask him, Mom."

"But he knows you."

"No, he doesn't. I just go in and buy sugar."

"Oh, please. Please do this for me, Poodie. It's only one day."

It was only one day. One day without sugar. But it would become one day of begging a favour from a stranger. Sitting at the kitchen table she put her head in her hands.

"Oh, my head," she sobs.

"Okay. I'll try."

Out the door, quietly down the wobbly wooden steps and around the corner to Niagara Street. A thousand tingles of fear ran up my back. I had never asked for credit before. How would I do it? It wasn't my idea. I'd have to make that clear. It was only one pound of ten cent sugar and only until tomorrow.

Then I'm standing at the long counter with the skinny old man looking down at me, waiting.

"My Mom asked me to ask you if she could have a pound of sugar and pay you the ten cents tomorrow."

There are his eyes. They're grey. They're dead. They're staring at me.

"No."

"She will pay you tomorrow."

"No."

Now what? He just stands there looking at me. The tingles of fear are now red flashes of embarrassment. So I leave, feeling his eyes on my back as I go. Mom is sitting at the kitchen table drinking tea.

"I'm sorry, Mom. He said no."

"Never mind. I borrowed a cup from the neighbour."

I never went back to the store beside the river.

* * *

"Hey, Freddie. What are you doing up in the middle of the night?"

I hadn't heard Paul come down the hall.

"Writing. I couldn't sleep."

"How can you see in here?" he asks.

"I can see . . . with the candle. But can you help me?"

"First, put on a sweater or something."

He takes his own jacket from the nail in the hallway and drapes it over me.

"Thanks."

"What do you need help with?" he asks.

"I think I want to write a poem about a ship. You know, an old schooner or a clipper."

Paul's interest piques, and he pulls out a chair from the table and sits next to me.

"Which is it? A schooner or a clipper?"

"Not sure."

"Okay. What do you need to know?"

"The different parts of a ship. What they're called."

"Do you mean the body of the ship like the keel or ribs? Or other parts like jibs, boom, topmasts?"

"I don't know. I want to say how beautiful it is, sailing across the waves like that. So free. Water splashing, wind blowing in the sails. But then maybe there's a storm and everything changes. So, what are the parts of the ship that would get crushed or wrecked?"

"When you say old do you mean eighteenth century?"

"I guess. Whenever sailing vessels were all there were."

"Well, let's say eighteenth century then."

"Okay."

Paul pulls his chair a little closer and takes a sheet of paper from the small pile I have on the table.

"Can I borrow your pencil?"

"Sure." And he begins to sketch.

"To begin with, the number of sails depends on what kind of sailing vessel you're talking about. It could be a three-mast schooner.

Or a brig with two masts or maybe a barque with three, four, or even five masts. But let's say it's a three-mast schooner."

For the next little while I am schooled in seafaring language while my brother radiates enthusiasm, sharing his love of all things nautical. He writes out the words I might want to use, and we talk about what would happen if a three-mast schooner was caught in a storm and crashed into the shore. I borrow the pencil back, and I scribble my thoughts down. When I look up at my brother's face, half lit in the candlelight, he's gazing into the distance of the dark room. I wonder if he's imagining the ship. I ask him,

"Do you think she sinks?"

"I think she must," he answers. "If she's got a huge rip below the water line there probably isn't much hope."

"So the ship is lost."

"Yes." He sounds melancholy at the loss of the imaginary vessel.

I put my pencil down and look at my page in the candlelight.

"One day we'll sail our own ship."

"Our own ship?" he asks turning to me.

"Our boat then. The one we're going to sail around the world. You and me. You remember."

"Oh. That boat."

"All around the world. We'll just go. You'll be Captain so we'll never crash and sink. I'll write a book all about it and we'll make a million dollars."

He laughs at my optimism. I laugh too.

"If you say so, Freddie."

"It's what we've always said we'd do."

"Yes. We did. You'd better get back to bed. One poem a night is enough."

"Aye aye, Captain!"

I pick up the sheet of paper and look over the words.

"Thanks for your help."

Warm hugs. Bare feet down the cold hallway to the front bedroom and back into bed with Jayne and Mom. They don't wake. He blows out the candle and sits for bit in the dark.

> She sails the blue as free as wind
> With cares of none to know,
> The sails, the mast, and spars, they bend
> As on the billows roll.
>
> She lends her sails to the mounting breeze
> As she clips o'er bounding waves,
> And finds her way through growing seas
> As the coming storm she braves.
>
> Now the rolling seas grow strong
> As o'er the decks they crash,
> The sky grows dark as the night bears on,
> And against her sail's winds lash.
>
> And now the ship she nears the rock,
> And now men lose control,
> And now she shudders with the shock
> As she runs upon the shoal.
>
> The seas pour in the mighty rip
> As on the reef she's tossed,
> Beneath the waves she starts to slip,
> And now the ship is lost.

*　　*　　*

You knew it was a special occasion if there was red pop. One bottle for Jayne. One bottle for me. Mom always had ginger ale. Three individual bags of chips and the party maker, French onion chip dip. New Years' Eve 1968. I couldn't wait for this year to begin. Come my next birthday I would finally be a teenager like Jayne. Your age had to have the word "teen" in it to be a teenager, Jayne had said. That didn't seem quite fair. After all she was only a year older. Well, a year and a bit. Fifteen months apart. That's how we were always described.

"No, not quite twins. Fifteen months apart."

But soon it wouldn't matter. In a few minutes, it would be 1969. Guy Lombardo would play Auld Lang Syne and Mom would cry like she always did. We would finish the last of our red pop, carefully sipped through the night to save enough for the toast, and I would be on my way to being a teenager. Finally.

Jayne sat on the edge of the lumpy red couch, fingering the tissue-wrapped gift we had cleverly hidden under it. A large, round glass pickle dish with three molded sections, secretly purchased at the Boxing Day sale from Woolworth's with the money Paul had sent home from Kapuskasing. He was living there and working on a chicken farm. Mom's birthday present. Next year maybe we'd fill it with crackers and cheese for New Years' Eve.

Only a minute to go now. Turn up the volume on the T.V. Now they're switching the broadcast to Times Square. The glittering ball was getting ready to fall. Any second now, and Ten! Nine! Eight! Pick up your pop. Here it comes. The seconds ticking into a completely new year. Pots would bang. The factory whistles would blow. Remember, Mom used to say that Dad was blowing that whistle on the years when he had to work this night. Somewhere on the edge of town a shotgun or two would blast in celebration. Three! Two! One! Happy New Year! Happy Birthday, Mom. She wrapped her arms around both of us and pulled us to herself so tightly that we were pushed face to face. And Mom was crying.

"Yes, yes. There won't be many more of these."

Wait. What? What was she saying? Jayne and I stared at each other, trying to decipher this new birthday celebration tradition.

"Next year, a new decade and then the Lord will come back. There won't be many more years after this."

Jayne rolled her eyes. But my breath caught in my throat and for the first of many times to come I felt the cold sweat of fear. But I'm just turning thirteen. I don't want it to end. Jayne pulled away from Mom's embrace.

"Here's your gift. Happy Birthday." She downed the last of her red pop and plopped onto the couch to watch revelry wash over Times Square.

*   *   *

"Fiona, get the Epsom salt. My feet are just killing me."

"Oh, for Christ's sake. If she wanted to call me Fiona, why did she name me Jayne?" That was something Jayne would never resolve.

Mom sank into the sagging red couch with an exhausted thump and lay her head back against the wall. There were some afternoons that just seemed to be endless. Endless counting, lifting, sorting, lifting newspapers while the rolling of the old press roared in her ear. Her left ear. That's the one that faced the press for hours every day while she laboured away lifting, sorting, counting. The cement floor in the circulation department of the old *Evening Tribune* was mercifully cool in summer and mercilessly cold in winter but always hard on your feet. And standing for hours on end without a break didn't help the pain in her varicose veins, that's for sure. But today it was her feet that ached. Wednesday. Insert day. All the ads for the local A&P, Loblaws, and Ford Dealerships went in the Wednesday insert and that made the papers even heavier.

It wasn't much of a job, but she was thankful for it. Thankful for the $14.50 a week and fearful of making any more. Family allowance penalized you for earning any more than that. It wouldn't have mattered if she had been working full-time somewhere. She wouldn't have needed Family Allowance, wouldn't have been subjected to the humiliation of it with all its rules and investigative visits. She would have had privacy, pride. That would have been grand. But who was going to hire a recently widowed fifty-year-old Bible school dropout? The circulation department of the *Evening Tribune*. That's who. Why look any further?

The awful truth that Mom would never know was that she was more talented than she gave herself credit for. She should have been, at the very least, working the front desk. At the very most, writing her own column. She had a memory like a steel-trap and could calculate figures in her head in the wink of an eye. A bundle of fifty less eighteen makes thirty-two for the Crowland/Dain City route. Fifty less twenty-two makes twenty-eight for Pelham.

Sometimes, the things she had learned by rote as a child or at Bible school kept her from falling into despair at the monotony of her job. "And Jacob sired Reuben and Simeon and Levi. Judah and Dan and so on. In the House of Normandy 1066 to 1087 William the First. 1087 to 1100 William the Second. Henry the First 1100 to 1135." And so on.

"Did you go to school this afternoon?" She asked Jayne.

"No."

"Oh, no! Did they call?"

Jayne hated it when Mom did that crying thing with her voice, as if she were terrified of the world and everything in it.

"I didn't answer the phone."

"But you'll go tomorrow?"

"I guess."

"Oh good."

"I'll need a note."

"What will I say? Were you sick?"

About bloody time she asked how I was feeling.

"No."

"Oh, dear."

If Jayne wasn't sick, what could she say? She couldn't lie. Lying was the greatest of all sins. And she couldn't say "My daughter refuses to go to school and I can't make her." That would be too embarrassing.

"Call it flu."

"And was it flu?"

"I guess."

"Oh, good."

There. Resolved.

Mom saw the oval, all-purpose basin half shoved under the couch where Jayne had been lying all day, watching TV.

"So, you weren't sick." Her sensibilities not allowing her to say the word vomit.

"No, I wasn't sick."

"Oh, good."

She pulled the basin fully out from under the red couch with her foot and slid it into the middle of the floor for Jayne to retrieve.

"Get the Epsom salt then, dear. My feet are killing me."

There was a time when Mom's feet didn't ache, when her legs were shapely and strong, and she was young enough to handle any hardship.

The front door pushed open with a loud complaint and I blew in, loaded with books.

"I'm home!" I called out.

Jayne stepped out of the kitchen where she was waiting for the kettle to boil.

"Where's Mom?"

Jayne cocked her head toward the living room.

"In there, talking to herself."

I put my books down on the dining room table and peeked around the corner and down the hall. Mom sat on the couch, her naked feet stretched out before her as though waiting to be anointed. Her eyes were closed, and her head was lifted toward Heaven. You could see her lips moving just a bit as she mumbled something to someone.

"Ah, she's praying." I concluded.

"If you say so."

"Did you go to school this afternoon?"

"Don't you start."

"Sorry, I just—"

"Yeah. Right."

Jayne grabbed her jacket from the board of nails next to the kitchen door and slid past me as the kettle began to boil.

"She wants Epsom salt."

She put her two hands on the front door and pulled. It took two hands to open it.

"Where are you going?"

"Out. See ya'."

She pulled the door shut behind her and ran down the steps. Mom would not like that.

"Don't pound on the stairs!" she would cry. "The neighbours will complain! Please!"

But no protest came.

I slid off my shoes, hung my coat on a nail and went to turn off the whistling kettle which Mom didn't seem to hear.

The thought of the mission fields in China still stirred an ache in her heart. She should have gone. She should have stayed the course. So many mistakes. So many wrong decisions.

"Oh, I'm sorry, Herb. I don't mean that we were a mistake. How could I have done anything but fall in love with you?" she half whispered to herself. "There really was no choice."

She heard his laughter first. Where was she? There was the distant sound of a plaintive train whistle. The light through her window had faded to purple and the tree that shaded her bedroom through warm September afternoons was a silhouette of black. How long had she slept? Oh, no. She's missed dinner again. Her hostess would not approve of that.

Now, laughter. Unexpected in this quiet house. Genuine and warm laughter from . . . from where? The kitchen. She smoothed her dress, her hair, her apprehension, and carefully dabbing a bit of perfume behind her ears, slowly walked down the back stairs to the kitchen. Warm light and the unfamiliar smell of tobacco filled the room. And laughter. Everyone was laughing. Ernie, Maggie, her mother and even Grandmother Rose.

Then he turned. He was tall and slender, his wavy hair combed neatly back off his handsome, sculpted face. Deep, piercing blue eyes and a perfectly trimmed moustache, slim like Errol Flynn. And lips which even from a distance seemed soft and welcoming in their winning smile. His clean, white cotton shirt was open just at the neck and tucked neatly into cuffed tweed trousers. In his large hands he held his fedora before him.

Grandmother Rose looked up, an uncharacteristic smile on her thin lips.

"Herb, this is our house guest, Cathy Smith. She is a student at the Faith Tabernacle Bible School in Toronto and sent to us by Sister Pennobecker for a bit of a holiday and a rest. Miss Smith, my very favourite nephew, Herbert Bray."

Taking a step forward and sweeping his hat to the side, he made a deep, courtly bow before her.

"It's a pleasure," he purred.

Maggie giggled, and her mother shushed her but continued to smile. Everyone seemed to be smiling.

You scoundrel. You facetious scoundrel. Is this some kind of joke or are you truly a gentleman? And do I want to know?

His eyes met hers and sparkled. He didn't seem to be mocking. But he was so out of place with what she had come to expect in this house. She would risk it.

"How do you do?" She offered her hand to shake.

Bowing again, he took her slender hand in his and kissed the back of it.

"Charmed."

Ernie blurted out a loud guffaw as young Rose gently slapped Herb on the back.

"Oh, Herbie, you're awful!"

Cathy snapped her hand back. She could feel the redness begin to tingle across her cheeks and up her neck to her ears. How dare they? How dare they embarrass her so?

"Rosie," he answered evenly, "I am in earnest. Don't laugh. My apologies, Miss Smith. Our good humour has gotten the best of us. It is truly a pleasure to meet you."

"Thank you." Now she didn't know what to think.

Grandmother Rose took control of the room once more.

"Herbert has paid us a surprise visit, Cathy. He has just dropped out of the sky after much too long an absence and has made this old woman very happy indeed."

Did she just call me Cathy?

Maggie jumped from her chair and threw her arms around Herb's waist.

"Herb is my very favourite, very distant cousin and I adore him!"

"Oh, brother." Ernie scoffed.

"Shut up, Ernie. You don't know anything."

Herb turned from Cathy, put an arm around the young girl and gave her a gentle squeeze.

"Well, thank you, Maggie. I adore you too."

"Madeline, set the table. Rose, reheat the chicken. Herb is hungry."

"Oh, Aunt Rose, I don't need a hot meal. Honestly. Just a sandwich."

"Nonsense. You've had a long day and you'll not leave here without a hot meal. Miss Smith slept through dinner. She will join you."

"Will you, Miss Smith?"

"Call me Cathy, please."

"Cathy. Please. Join me for dinner."

"I don't mind. Thank you."

"It's a pleasure." And he bowed again.

Grandmother Rose gave his arm a gentle slap.

"Oh, Herbert. For heaven's sake. Enough shenanigans. Go sit in the living room and put your feet up."

"Yes, Aunt Rose." This time he bowed to her.

"Oh, go on you nut."

"Cathy?" He offered his arm.

She took it, still not knowing if she was part of the joke or the brunt of it. And yet he seemed very much in earnest, placing his hand over hers to lead her through to the burgundy and mahogany living room.

Grandmother Rose snapped at Maggie as they left the kitchen.

"Not in here, child. Set the dining room table. The dining room."

Herb took a deep breath and smiled.

"Hmm. Evening in Paris."

"Yes."

Cathy could feel the young girl's cold stare follow them as they walked together out of the room.

Their first date was a few days later. The Welland Fair. Their second date was a picnic in a park beside the canal. Not his favourite kind of meal but Cathy's idea of romance—a throwback to the picnics of her adolescence. A movie at the Capitol Theatre. A walk through Chippewa Park. And all too soon for them both, her visit to Welland ended. But their courtship had just begun. Throughout the fall, past Christmas and into the New Year they would write to each other and rendezvous whenever possible, most often in Hamilton, the halfway distance between their lives.

On the last day of January, he had made up his mind.

"Cathy, I love you and you're going to marry me."

"Is that a proposal?"

"Yes. Let's get married."

"When?"

"Next week."

"Next week! I can't."

"Why not?" "

"Well, I need to tell Sister Pennobecker and ask her to marry us. I need a dress. We need a place to live!"

"All right. The week after, then. You find the dress and I will find the place to live. Where is my pocket calendar?"

He pulled the small paper calendar from his wallet and looked at the date.

"Two weeks today is . . . February 14."

"Valentine's Day."

"That settles it. Two weeks today, Cathy. We'll be married anywhere you like but we will be married on Valentine's Day."

And that was that.

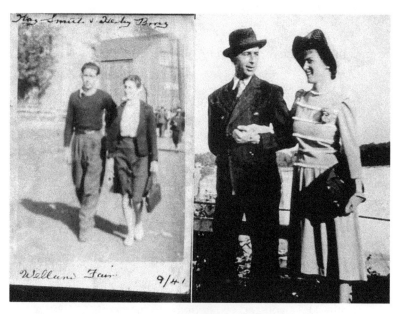

First date at Welland Fair (1941), left.
Newlyweds in Niagara Falls, Ontario (1942), right.

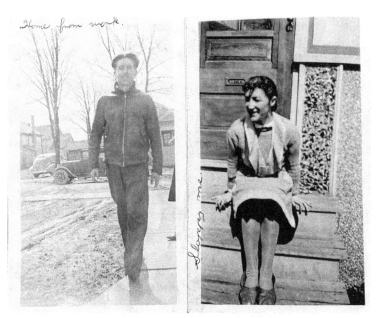

Herb home from work (1942), left.
Cathy waiting on the steps in the sun (1942), right.

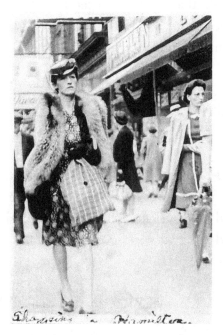

The fashionable Mrs. Bray shopping in Hamilton (1943)

"Mom?"

Who was that, now?

"Mom, are you awake?"

"Oh. Yes, I'm awake. Just resting my eyes."

"You didn't drink your tea."

"Oh. Thank you, dear."

She takes a large gulp from the teacup on the coffee table.

"Ach. Stone cold. Make another pot, Poodie, please."

"Sure, Mom."

I go into the kitchen and turn the kettle back on. She calls to me from the living room. "Where's your sister?"

"She went out."

"Of course she did. I need you to go to the A&P."

"What for? I have homework."

"Bread and sugar."

"Okay."

I'm fairly certain that we'll soon need tea as well.

"What are your plans, Poodie?"

"I have St. John's Ambulance tonight."

"What time?"

"6:30."

It's always 6:30 but I have to tell her that every week.

"Well, you'd better go to the A&P right away."

"I will."

"There's a two-dollar bill in my purse. Take that."

Mom's brown handbag is on the couch next to her. I click open the top latch and take out her change purse to find the orange two-dollar bill, folded in half. I stick it into the pocket of my pants.

"Poodie, the kettle is boiling."

"I know."

I turn off the kettle, make the tea, and deliver the whole pot to her before heading out the door.

"And don't pound on the stairs. Please!"

"I won't." I never do.

She swishes the warm water in the plastic, oval basin and rubs one foot over the other, gently massaging her crooked toes. Her poor, unsightly, crooked toes. Closing her eyes again she begins to drift.

"Cathy, time to get up. Wake up, dear."

Jessie pushed the heavy curtains aside to begin the day. The early morning amber poured in through the large bedroom window, but Cathy didn't stir. Her little girl seemed so tiny, so precious in her small bed.

"Cathy?" She pushed the long braid away from the child's neck and ran her hand across her forehead to try and rouse her. Hot! She was so hot! "Dear God, she's burning up. Jim!" Even her frantic call didn't stir the child.

"Jim! Come quick!"

He appeared in the bedroom doorway, still buttoning his shirt. "What is it?"

"She's burning up! I can't wake her."

"Calm down, Jessie. It may be nothing. Let me see." He sat on the edge of the bed and gently stroked his daughter's head. "Cathy girl. It's Daddy. Wake up, dear."

"Oh God. Dear God."

"Jessie! Calm down. You'll only frighten her. Now calm down."

He turned his attention back to his child, stroking her cheek now and speaking gently as though softly calling her from a long distance. "Cathy. Cathy, girl. Time to wake up."

"Daddy?" Her own voice a crackling whisper, she opened her eyes but didn't seem to focus.

"Yes, dear. It's Daddy. Are you awake?"

"My throat hurts."

Jessie broke the calm. "She's caught something from those nasty children. I told you she shouldn't be playing with those nasty, dirty children."

"Jessie! Enough." Somewhere between angry and terrified, Jessie backed into the corner of the room and watched as her husband calmed the child with matter-of-fact conversation. "You've slept a little late this morning, Cathy."

"It's itchy, Daddy. Itchy."

"Where, dear. Show Daddy where it itches."

She tugged at the buttons down the front of her flannelette night gown. "Here."

Carefully, he unbuttoned the nightie at her neck, then down her chest. He took her hand and pushed the long sleeve up one arm, turning it to examine it in the pale morning light. Then just as calmly he tucked her under her blanket and stroked her head. "Alright now. Mother will get you a drink of water and you try to take a sip or two. All right?"

"All right."

"Good Girl. Jessie, call the doctor. Tell him we may need an ambulance."

"An ambulance! Why? What is it?"

"I think it may be scarlet fever."

The doctor arrived and then the ambulance. The whispers in the street floated mournfully up to the windows of their second floor flat. The dreaded phrase. Scarlet Fever. Poor thing. So young. Poor Jessie. She'll never recover from losing that child. Poor thing. Poor, poor thing.

"No, Mommy. I don't want to go in the ambulance. I don't want to!" Cathy clutched the blanket to her face and shrank as deeply as she could into her pillow, coughing and crying with the pain.

"There's nothing to be afraid of. It will be a great adventure, riding in an ambulance."

"I don't want to. No! No! No!"

"Cathy. Stop it now, for heaven's sake!" But her mother's insistence only caused the child to painfully sob even more. Jessie turned to her husband, frustration and near defeat in her face.

Then he sat on the bed and wiped the tears from Cathy's red cheeks.

"What are you afraid of, dear? Tell Daddy."

"People die in ambulances."

"Who told you that?" he asked her with a smile.

"Georgina. Georgina said ambulances come when people die. I don't want to die, Daddy. Don't make me."

"Listen dear. The ambulance is here to take you to the hospital where they will make you better. You don't think your mother and I would send you in an ambulance if it would hurt you, do you?"

"No," she whispered, not quite convinced.

Her mother chimed in, cajoling her.

"Besides, Cathy. An ambulance ride will be fun."

"What are you telling her?" Jim barely concealed his frustration with his wife. But the lie calmed the child.

"Fun?" she wanted to know.

"Yes, dear." her mother continued. "You'll have all kinds of good things in the ambulance."

"Like what?"

"Oh, music. Candy and books."

"Jessie," his voice warned.

"Books?" That was something Cathy loved.

"Yes," she said. "You are a lucky little girl, getting to ride in an ambulance. Everyone will watch you and say, 'What a lucky little girl.'"

"They will?"

"Of course."

"Okay. I'll go," the child conceded.

"There, now. That's my good girl." Jessie lifted the blankets from the child, but Jim stepped forward, moving her aside.

"I'll take her. Come with Daddy, dear."

He gathered his little girl in his arms and took her through to the living room where two burly orderlies in white coats and heavy boots waited. At the side of the stretcher stood a crisply starched and unsmiling nurse. To Cathy she was a blur of white, floating toward her in a waft of antiseptic air.

"I'll take her from here." the nurse declared as she lifted Cathy out of her father's arms. Then laying her on the stretcher, the nurse covered her with a grey blanket, secured two straps across her small body and nodded to the orderlies. They carried Cathy down the stairs and past the neighbours, whose sad eyes peaked above the hankies and scarves they held over their mouths and noses. Scarlet fever, they murmured, shaking their heads in premature grief. Poor thing. Poor, poor thing.

The small gathering of onlookers parted to make way. Tucked beneath the protective arms of their parents, Cathy's playmates watched as she passed by, bundled under the blanket on the stretcher. Some were silently weeping, others sadly waving her goodbye from a short safe distance. And there was Georgina stepping back and shaking her head. None of them seemed envious of the lovely ride Cathy was going to have.

She turned her head away from her friends to see the bright, red cross painted on the side of the vehicle. The ambulance where books and music and toys waited. Except that they didn't. As they slid her headfirst into the back of the dark canvass-covered vehicle, no music played. No candy was offered, and no toys appeared.

"Where are they?" she asked the nurse, who was seating herself on the opposite side of the truck. "Where are they?" Cathy repeated, forcing an answer.

"Your parents are not allowed to ride in the ambulance."

"The books. The music."

"She all right?" asked one of the orderlies as he climbed into the back.

"Just the fever talking. She'll sleep soon."

"Right." The orderly settled back against the side of the truck, pulled a mask over his mouth and nose, and crossed his arms against his chest as the ambulance lurched forward, grinding its gears toward the hospital.

Something wasn't right. Her mother had said there would be books and music. But she had lied. How could she when lying was the greatest of all sins? She had lied and sinned. Why? Nothing made sense to the child. Maybe she was going to die after all.

"It's all right dear," whispered the nurse as she wiped a tear from Cathy's cheek. "You sleep now. We'll be there soon, and everything will be all right."

But it wasn't going to be all right. Mother had lied and now they were taking her away in an ambulance to die. I don't want to die. I don't want to die.

"Hush now. Hush. No one is going to die."

Sleep pulled her, unwillingly, into a void as the ambulance jostled along the narrow streets away from home.

"I'm back!"

There is no answer from the living room, and I wonder if Mom has drifted off to sleep. I can see her from the end of the hall. She's still sitting on the couch, eyes closed, with her feet in the basin. That water must be cold by now. But maybe it feels good. It's an unusually hot autumn afternoon. Which means it's a typically hot apartment, and the curtains on both windows are open to the afternoon sun. I close them, open a window a bit to let in a breeze, and say to Mom, "Is that better? Do you feel cooler now?"

She stirs without opening her eyes. "It's all right, dear."

I pull the change from the grocery store out of my pocket and return it to her purse. Nickels, dimes, and quarters.

Now a cool feeling across her hot brow. A cloth. Someone was laying a cool cloth on her forehead. She opened her eyes. A white blur drifted beside her. She wasn't in the ambulance anymore. Where was she? Now a soft hand and gentle voice, "Hello little one."

Was it an angel?

"Am I dead? Who?" The words scratched her throat. She coughed then whimpered in pain.

The angel smiled soothingly.

"No sweetheart. Of course not. Lie still now. It's all right, dear."

"Who?" The words came too painfully to finish the question.

"I'm a nurse, and I'm here to help you. Everything is all right."

The angel nurse rinsed the cloth in more cool water then lay it again across Cathy's burning brow.

"That's better now, isn't it?"

It was better. But different. Everything was different. This wasn't her nightgown. This wasn't her bed. And where was Daddy?

Jim and Jessie walked on foot to the hospital. By the time they arrived, Cathy had been admitted, examined, and ensconced within the isolation ward. The doctor stood with them in the hall just outside the doors to the ward where their little girl lay. He spoke quietly, saying the words he had so frequently spoken of late to other parents in this same hallway.

"As you know, there is no cure, only treatment."

"I am aware." Sergeant Major James Smith had seen diseases like this firsthand in the trenches and was all too familiar with the facts.

"But we can make her quite comfortable. We'll keep her hydrated and cool until the fever breaks."

Jessie spoke up. "Will she scar? Will the red marks scar her?"

"Possibly. We'll monitor the rash, Mrs. Smith, and if necessary, cover her hands with gloves to prevent scratching. She will require complete bed rest in the isolation ward for a number of weeks. After that time, if she responds well to treatment and is strong enough, she may be able to begin taking meals in the common dining room. There are possible side effects with scarlet fever, of course. A weakened heart, possible kidney disorder, mobility issues. It's possible that she will recover fully with no other issues. But only time will tell. That is all I can say at this point in time."

"May we see her to say goodbye?" Jim asked.

"I'm afraid not. Contagions, you understand. Only medical personnel in the isolation ward. Perhaps when she is moved to another ward you will be able to visit. As I said, that is all I can tell you at this time."

"Thank you." Jim took Jessie's hand and lay it in the crook of his arm. They walked home together.

Feet together she gently splashed them in and out of the plastic basin. The soreness would eventually pass. It always did. But the crumpled toes would be the same. Battle scars. Souvenirs from a time when loneliness was a state of being. Books were the solitary friends. Breakfast was buttermilk and tinctures, and the only learning to take place was that of how to walk again once the disease had crippled her feet, seemingly for life.

*   *   *

Their voices had begun low and quiet behind the closed kitchen door but now I can hear them all the way down the hall. Paul is there too. I'm the only one outside of the conversation.

Jayne is arguing with Mom.

"We're just going to go to City Hall or something and get married."

"Why so quickly? Do you have to?"

I have to get out of here, was the answer that ran through Jayne's head, but she knew what Mom meant. Did she "have to" because she was pregnant?

"No. I don't 'have to.'"

"Then there is no need to rush. Finish school," Mom said, definitively.

"I *am* finished school. I'm sixteen and now I can quit."

"Where will you live?"

"His brother has a house that we can rent a room in."

I could hear my sister's determination. Her mind was made up.

"I don't even know this boy." Mom said.

"He's not a boy. He's a man."

"How old?"

"As old as Jim was when he got married."

"Paul, tell her she's too young."

"Paul?" Jayne sounds not only plaintive but defiant, her strong suit.

"If you want to quit school, you can. You're old enough," our brother replied. "But you need Mom's permission to marry."

"I KNOW! That's the only reason I told her. I just wanted to run away but Pat said we had to ask you."

If they're going to get married anyway, why doesn't she just agree to wait, I wonder? Does she really hate it at home all that much? My logic seems sound. I open the door to the kitchen, walk in, and stand by the sink. Everyone is standing.

"Can I just say something?" I offer.

Three voices in unison turn on me. "No!"

"This has nothing to do with you," Mom adds.

Then Paul softens the blow.

"It's all right, Freddie. Just go back in the living room and watch T.V."

The arguing continues as Paul closes the kitchen door behind me with a smile.

"I didn't even want to get married," I hear Jayne say.

"Then why are you?"

"Because *he* wants to. He won't just live with me. It's against his religion."

"What's his religion?" Mom asks, somewhat alarmed.

I think I can hear my sister's voice starting to break. If she starts crying now Jayne will be furious with herself, I know. Hers will be tears of anger and frustration, but Mom won't see them that way. Then Paul's voice defuses the room.

"Come on, Jayne, Mom. Let's all sit down."

Three chairs scrape across the kitchen linoleum and the room returns to muted tones behind the closed door. Paul is saying something. I don't hear the words anymore, but I do hear his voice calming Jayne. They talk a long while. Questions. Acquiescence. The sound of light laughter muted in a hug. Finally, the kitchen door opens and I see Jayne wrapped in Paul's arms, standing in the doorway.

"Okay?" he asks softly.

"Okay," she answers.

He gives a small laugh.

"Sure. It'll be fine. You'll see."

The open door is an invitation for me to join the rest of the family, I think.

"You okay?" I ask Jayne.

"She's fine," Mom answers for her. "And guess what? We're going to have a wedding in June!"

"Really? Jaynie! You're getting married in June?"

"Yeah. Yeah, I am."

She squeezes my arm as she passes me in the doorway and heads down to the bedroom.

"Wow. A wedding. Well that just leaves you and me, eh Paul?"

He says nothing but smiles and looks at Mom and says, "Well, not necessarily."

His look is either cautious or apologetic. Maybe both.

"What do you mean?"

"I won't be here."

Then he decides to tell me.

"I'm getting married, too."

My brain goes numb.

"What? No. We're supposed to sail around the world together. What about the plan? Our plan?"

"I'm sorry, Freddie. Things don't always work out the way you plan."

"But you can't be leaving too. You can't!"

"But I am. I'm getting married in January."

"To who?"

"You don't know her."

Married. In January. To a stranger. I can't understand it. I can't understand it at all. We're supposed to travel together. See the world . . . together. I'm going to write a book.

"Two weddings in one year." Mom has perked up. "And then it will be just you and me, Poodie."

Everybody knew. Everybody knew except me. That's why Jayne will wait until June. Paul is getting married first. And everybody knew. And now it will just be Mom and me.

Now he hugs me and chuckles softly as I cry.

"Oh, Freddie. Don't. Don't."

My heart sinks, pushed down through the floorboards by heavy sorrow, fear, and an inexplicable sense of betrayal.

* * *

"Good morning, and welcome. My name is Robert Wright here at C-HOW Radio in Welland with our regular programme sponsored by the Clergy Fellowship."

Robert rarely introduced himself as Reverend Wright of All Peoples' United. Saying "Reverend" put some people off. Made them feel self-conscience and uncomfortable. Then you couldn't really talk with them, listen to them, and truly understand who they really were. Still, most people who lived in Welland knew who Robert Wright was. The outspoken, rebellious pastor of the people and all things related to the common good and peace on Earth. You know, like Jesus.

"I would like to welcome back a frequent and always enjoyable guest to our programme, Kay Bray. Welcome, Kay."

"Thank you, Robert."

"Kay, for those who don't know you, you are not an ordained minister, but you frequently pinch hit for some of us when called upon to take a service. You have taken the pulpit for Evangelistic Healing Missions, the Salvation Army Citadel, open air services and, of course, All Peoples' United. In fact, you were kind enough to take the service for me at Chaffey Street All Peoples' this past week in spite of the fact that you are nursing a sprained ankle. Is that right, Kay?"

"Oh, yes. But that doesn't hold me back."

"So I've heard. More than one person told me that it was the best one-legged sermon they ever heard!"

They laugh together, and she gently slaps his forearm in appreciation. It's good to be appreciated.

"Well, I know that your messages are inspiring and dramatic. Even theatrical. And of course, that's the way it's supposed to be!"

"Absolutely." She agrees.

"And you are also quite an activist. I remember the first CCF meeting I ever attended. It was at your home on State Street. You and your husband hosted. How does that kind of work jive with your ministry?"

"Well, some of my Pentecostal friends chide me for my involvement in the Peace Movement, the CCF and now the NDP. I don't see any conflict in being a Christian and also a social activist. They should go hand in hand. People tell me, `You can't bring in the

Rapture until after Armageddon.' But I say, no, but there is nothing wrong with trying to make the world a better place now."

"Kay, are you a Jesus freak?"

"We've been friends for a long time," she replies with a sly smile.

"Really?' Robert dares to ask, "How long?"

"All my life. And that is a good many years."

They laugh, good naturedly, and Robert pursues the thought.

"Tell us more, Kay."

"Are you sure you want me to? Some people say I talk too much."

"Please, Kay. I'm sure our listeners want to hear."

And he wants to know more. So, she shares with all of Welland a history she has not even told her children. It begins to explain so much.

"I was an only child and didn't really have any friends."

"You? Had no friends? I find that hard to believe." Robert knows Kay Bray to be gregarious and outgoing.

"No, it's true. Mother did not approve of most other children. They were dirty or ill-mannered. They were not `our kind,' whatever that meant. `Stick to your own kind' she would say. So, when I was little it was my Grandmother Stewart I spent time with. Granny liked going places and so we went! The zoo and the seaside and parks, Granny and I went. We were real pals. But a Granny is not a playmate."

"No, I suppose not." Robert agrees.

"No. So I took to myself a secret friend. However, this was not just an imaginary friend. I had Jesus. I loved Him, talked to Him, I told Him everything. If I wanted to go shopping or to the theatre, I asked Him. I was rather afraid of God. He was intimidating. But not Jesus."

"And that was when you became friends?"

"Yes. I visited with him often, especially on Sundays. In Edinburgh, at St. Ninians, I went to Church at eleven. I went back to Sunday school at 2:00 pm. Then into another church service at

3:00 pm. Back to church at seven at night, into the church hall at eight for Evangelistic service and then out into the street for street meeting at nine."

"Talk about going to church!" Robert laughs.

"Well, I had no time to be bored. It was just as well for I was not allowed to pick up a toy or a book on the Sabbath."

"You mentioned the Evangelical Service. Was St. Ninians a Pentecostal Church?"

"No. Presbyterian. Church of Scotland."

"When did you become Pentecostal, then?"

"Oh, that was when we moved to Bathurst, New Brunswick. A new preacher came to town to preach the Gospel in the Masonic Hall and that started the Pentecostal Church in Bathurst."

"Some of our listeners may not understand the difference between Presbyterian and Pentecostal, Kay. How are they different, in your experience?"

"Well, they are different in the way we worship, I suppose. You can really get caught up in the liveliness of a Full Gospel meeting. Everybody sings. Everybody praises Jesus right out loud. It can be very invigorating. Perhaps not so much these days. But in those years, in my youth, we really knew what it was to be Pentecostals. And it was not always easy to be one."

"What do you mean?" Robert asks.

"We were called Holy Rollers, although I never did see anyone roll. We were laughed at all the time. We never cut our hair, we never wore make up, and always wore dark stockings. In other words, we really dressed our part."

Robert smiles and then says, "When you say you were laughed at, didn't that disturb you? Make you feel like an outcast?"

"Sometimes. But being apart, separate from others, was nothing new to me. Besides, it brought us closer together as a fellowship. And remember, I was never really alone."

"Because of your secret friend that makes you a Jesus Freak?"

"I told you. We have been friends a long time." She smiles with satisfaction and a private, spiritual pride.

*   *   *

I had just started high school. Grade nine. But everyone else seemed to be getting married! First Paul then Jayne. Then Jayne's new in-laws, Rose, then Dianne. And now my childhood friend, Thiel. Within twelve months I was in four bridal parties, and I didn't even have a boyfriend. That was my lament as I visited Mrs. Gorbet one afternoon.

Few teachers would have taken the time outside of school to enrich a student's understanding and curiosity. But Mrs. Gorbet did. On the last day of grade four, standing outside the school in the sun, she had told me that even though she was changing schools and would not be at Queen Street anymore she would like to keep in touch. Maybe I could visit her home, with my mother's permission of course. Would I like that? Would I continue to share my poems with her? Visit a teacher outside of school! That had never happened before. But I said yes and so did Mom.

And so, Mrs. Gorbet welcomed me and my scribblings into her home. And scribblings they were. Naive writings about Nature or God. Little love poems or odes to broken hearts. She was always so patient and praising of my efforts. So was her husband, Frank. Mrs. Gorbet had become a guiding light in my often unsure existence, and I visited frequently.

On one of those days, when she and Frank had recently returned from New York City, she sat me down in the den and handed me an album cover.

"Read this as you listen," she said.

Then she put on the New York recording of Fiddler on the Roof and went into the kitchen, leaving me alone. For two hours, I sat in their den listening and reading as the story unfolded in my mind's eye. That was my introduction to Broadway. It was fantastic.

But on this particular day it wasn't poetry, theatre, or cinema that concerned me. It was the fact that everyone else seemed to be getting married and I didn't even have a boyfriend. I was in high school!

"Are you jealous of that?" she asked me.

"I don't know." And I didn't.

"Listen to me," she said. "Some of your friends may very well marry before you do. They will quit school, get a job, and start a new life. But what kind of life will it be without an education, without life experience? What kind of jobs or careers can they have? And remember this. It is hard to be romantic at the end of the day when the bills aren't paid."

*   *   *

PART THREE

L'AMOUR

We are drinking tea, of course. We're using her Royal Albert teacups. Mom loves her new apartment in the seniors' building. It's small but warm and has a lovely little balcony overlooking the canal. She has put a small table and two chairs out here and we are sitting leisurely, drinking tea.

"When my mother died, I pulled out all the good linen, china and crystal for Dad and I and we used it every day. She never wanted to use it." Mom shares.

"She didn't? Why not?"

"She was saving it, I suppose. For what, I don't know. My wedding, maybe."

"But she didn't live long enough to see you and Dad married, did she?"

"Heavens, no. She died in 1936. That was when I met my Scotchman. We were engaged to be married the next year. But she died before that."

"But you didn't marry him, your Scotchman."

"No. Somehow I couldn't forget the one man I met when I broke my first engagement."

"Wait. You mean the fellow you met at church when you were sixteen?'

"I broke that engagement, too."

"Then who was the man you couldn't forget?'

She smiles. "My Frenchman."

This is news to me. "What was his name, Mom?"

She drifts into a kind of reverie now, a private world that she visits more and more frequently these days. Now she's somewhere else, remembering.

We weren't supposed to meet.

"Stick to your own kind," Mother said.

It's Sunday. I'm on the way home from my church. He has just come out of his. Why is he looking at me?

"Excusez-moi, Mademoiselle."

"Oh, hello."

"Bonjour."

"Bonjour."

Look how his deep brown eyes light up. "Ah! Parlez-vous Francais?'

"No."

"Ah, mais oui. Tu parles Francais."

"I'm sorry. I don't really speak French. I am British. Scottish."

"Mais vous me parlez Français. Oui?"

"Juste un peu. Just a word here and there."

He is smiling. Is he making fun of me? No. It's a lovely smile.

"Moi, aussi. Je parle un peu l'Anglais."

"English? You speak a little English?"

"Oui. Je te parlerai en Francais et tu me parleras en Anglais. C'est bon?"

"I'm not sure what you said, but I think I understand you."

"Oui. On se comprends entre nous." (We understand each other)

I do understand him. Somehow, I feel that I know him. Or I want to know him. He's stepping closer.

"Belle Écossaise. Nous allons apprendre de l'un et l'autre."
(Beautiful Scottish girl. We will teach each other.)

I don't know what he's saying. Maybe we can teach other. Yes. I think we will.

"Mom?"

"Hmmm?"

"What was his name, your Frenchman?"

"Jean. His name was Jean."

"You loved him."

"I should have. But then I wouldn't have you, would I?"

"But you did love him."

"It was quite romantic for a while." She smiles. "A group of us would go to Tetagouche Falls to picnic and swim, and he would just be there. Or we would meet in secret. There, or somewhere else in town. Oh, he was something, my Jean. I believe I broke his heart."

"You broke up with him?"

"My people would not have approved. He was French. And Catholic. But I wish I had been braver. I wish someone had said to me 'Don't let race or background or relatives or friends come between you and the one you love. Follow your heart.' That's good advice, Poodie. Follow your heart."

I don't know what to say. I'm trying to imagine my mother, my seventy-year-old mother as a young, rebellious, girl falling in love with her handsome Frenchman. A forbidden love. Well, she wasn't always seventy years old, you know.

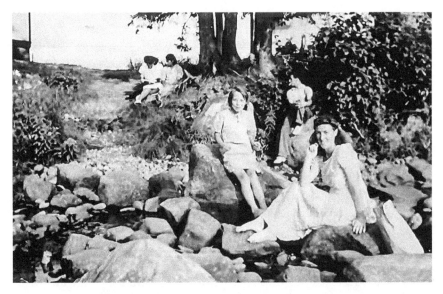

Young Cathy Smith at Tetagouche Falls, New Brunswick
(Is that Jean in the background?)

*   *   *

He came by it naturally. That's what Mom always said. Dad had a green thumb, and he came by it naturally.

The five potted African violet plants in Jayne's front window were thriving. They sat side by side, perfectly spaced, each one independent of the other yet still creating one flawless window garden. True to their name, their blooms were a deep violet colour and they nestled cozily amid their soft, rounded leaves. Jayne was rightfully proud of her plants and her home.

I had driven Mom up to Hamilton to visit my sister and see the house that she and her family had recently bought. A home. Finally, in a home of her own, Jayne glowed with delight and obvious contentment. She ushered us from room to room, showing off each one, highlighting their unique Victorian attributes. The long front hall that ran the near length of the house. The living room window that looked out onto the large, shaded veranda. Her dining room, separated from the front room by the fine latticework arch. The wooden banister and newel post that led to the second floor. Hardwood throughout. And at the back of the house, her kitchen. Her large, eat-in kitchen where she would create delicious, miraculous meals for her family. Delicious because she could make anything. Miraculous because she often did it with next to nothing. Everything about the house thrilled her. And if anyone could make a house into a home, it was Jayne.

"Do you think we could have a cup of tea, Fiona?" Mom asked Jayne, as she collapsed onto the couch.

"Don't you want to go to lunch?" I asked.

"Yes, oh yes. But let's have a cup of tea first. Please."

We recognized the tone of Mom's voice, a kind of exhaustion that bordered on pleading. We would have tea first.

"I'll help." I told my sister. We left Mom reclining on the couch, eyes closed, and feet outstretched. As I glanced back into the living room I appreciated, again, Jayne's beautiful African violets.

"I don't know how you do it, Jaynie. Your plants are lovely. Just like Dad's used to be. Do you remember them on the sill of our dining room bay window?"

"Oh, yeah." She smiled. "He had a real green thumb."

He came by it naturally, his green thumb. That's what Peter and Minnie told Cathy when she had first met them at their farm. What a day that was, she remembered.

Spending time with Herb had been lovely. He was such a gentleman and seemed to genuinely enjoy her company. Their days together had obviously become dates, and he did his best to make them memorable.

As they strolled through Chippewa Park one day, Cathy commented on the beautiful roses and said how she missed having a garden like the one back home in Bathurst.

"You love Nature, don't you?" he asked her. "Living in Toronto, you must miss it."

"Yes," Cathy answered with a small sigh. "I love all of God's natural world. I really enjoy Toronto, but I also love where your aunt lives. It's wonderful to wake up to the sound of birds again."

"Would you like to come with me tomorrow to our friends' farm? I have some planting to do, but you could wander about on your own if you like. Or help me. Whatever you please."

"That sounds like a lovely day. Where is their farm? Is it near your father's house?"

"No. It's the other direction. North of here. More than an hour on foot but not far by trolley. We would walk as far as the hospital and get the trolley from there, about a twenty-minute ride. Then it's just a mile or two to their farm. Would you like to come?"

"Absolutely. Thank you!" Cathy beamed.

"I'll come for you at eight then?"

"Don't come all the way to your aunt's house just to turn around and go back again. I can meet you at the top of River Road."

"Absolutely not. I will pick you up at eight. Wear walking shoes." He winked.

I brought the tray with the tea pot and mugs out to Jayne's dining room table, and called to Mom, "Here's the tea."

But she didn't move from the couch. I saw her lips moving, as they often did when she rested. Probably praying, I guessed.

Back in the kitchen, Jayne poured milk into a small pitcher and I grabbed the sugar. Can't have tea without sugar.

Herb and Cathy got off the trolley at Stop 17 and walked east along Quaker Road. It was a beautifully warm autumn day. In the woods to their left a gentle breeze floated through the trees.

Birds chirped and there was a distant sound of rustling, as though some wildlife was foraging in the forest.

"It's not too far," he assured her.

"Oh, I don't mind. I like to walk," she answered with a smile.

Soon they came to a break in the trees and a narrow, mud lane that led into the forest.

"This way, Cathy. Watch for ruts in the road."

Shifting the paper bag he carried to his left hand, he offered her his other one for assistance.

The lane was straight for the most part, but the trees formed a canopy above them that dappled the sunlight and sometimes obscured whatever may be in the distance. Goldfinches and robins chirped above.

A white, two-storey house came into view. It boasted a wide porch that covered what appeared to be two front doors. The lane ended at the front yard, a sea of dandelions that greeted them like a golden welcome mat.

Herb called out, "Hello the house!"

From the barn, a tall, lanky man in overalls and brimmed hat appeared, pitchfork in hand, and ambled toward them. As he walked, he called out.

"Minnie, come out. Herb is here!"

They heard a screen door banging, and from behind the house appeared a short, stout woman in a cotton dress, wiping her hands on her full calico apron. With the back of her hand, she pushed wisps of hair from her forehead and squinted into the sun.

"Herb?" she called. "You're late for breakfast. We'll have lunch. Who's that with ya?"

Herb smiled at Cathy and said, "Come on."

He led her across the dandelion carpet to be introduced.

"Minnie, Peter, this is Cathy Smith. She is staying with Aunt Rose in town and has come out today for a visit and some country air. Cathy, Minnie and Peter Zavitz, old family friends."

"Say now," Peter protested, "Not that old. Still baling my own hay."

Herb laughed.

"Hello, Cathy," Minnie said.

"Hello. So nice to meet you both," Cathy replied.

Taking his hat off his head and wiping his brow with his forearm, Peter turned toward the house.

"Well, come on in. Have some cold water. You'll be parched. Minnie, pump some fresh."

In the cool of their front room, Cathy learned the story of the Zavitz family, mostly from Herb because Minnie and Peter were people of few words. They were brother and sister and had emigrated from Europe with their parents in the early 1900s. They had owned and worked this farm ever since.

"They knew my dad before he married my mother," Herb explained. "Dad worked for Minnie and Peter's parents."

"Yup," said Peter.

Minnie nodded and said, "Percy. He has a green thumb, that one. Came to help on the farm."

"Like Herb, here," Peter added.

"Yup," Minnie agreed. "You got your dad's green thumb. Come by it naturally."

"Dad says hello," Herb told them. "He's sent you some daffodil bulbs, Minnie."

He showed her the paper bag he had set on the floor.

"I'm obliged," Minnie answered.

"I'll plant them for you today. Where would you like them?" Herb asked.

"Up to you."

"How about in front of the house?"

"Up to you."

Peter stood and put his hat on his head.

"Got work to do."

And he left by the back door, heading to the barn.

Minnie stood, picked up the mugs they had been drinking water from and went into the kitchen without a word.

Cathy looked at Herb, puzzled at the abrupt exits. He smiled and explained.

"It's just their way. I had better get these bulbs in the ground though."

"Would it be all right if I just walked about?"

"Of course. I'll look for you when it's lunch time. Enjoy."

"Thank you."

Minnie nodded in her direction as Cathy went through the kitchen and out the back door. A huge field lay before her stretching back to a thick stand of trees. In the field were two black and white cows and a brown horse, all quietly grazing. A perfect place to walk and pray.

Someone spoke.

"Your tea."

Who was that?

"Mom," Jayne said again. "Your tea is getting cold."

"Oh. Thank you."

Mom got up and walked into the dining room where Jayne and I were finishing our tea. She sat down and poured herself a cup from Jayne's china tea pot. Topping it up with milk and adding two spoons full of sugar, she stirred while looking off into some distance.

"Where are we going for lunch?" Jayne wanted to know.

"Mom wants to go to Tiffany's in Hess Village," I said.

"Really? That's great." My sister was excited. "Thanks, Mom."

But Mom did not reply, so I spoke to her too.

"Mom, we should go soon if we want to get a patio table."

That seemed to rouse her.

"Oh, yes. I love Tiffany's. And I'm starving."

"We'll go as soon as you finish your tea," I suggested.

Taking a sip, she predictably said, "Ach. No, let's just go. It's gone cold."

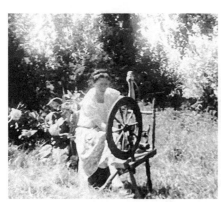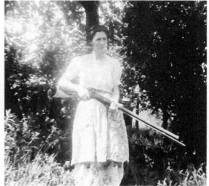

Cathy posing with antiques at the Zavitz's farm.

*   *   *

Sipping Brandy at forty thousand feet. Life is good. We follow the sun so that it seems to never set. Held by some invisible tie it pulls us around the horizon with it, following its path around the world. A wash of golden-brown clouds rests upon the line of the sky, here above the clouds. It fades into the blue light above it, reminding us that the sun shines just out of our reach. Time stands still as we chase the time master and I wonder what they're doing down there. There where the lights define the boundaries. I used to look up at planes passing overhead and try to imagine where people were going. Used to wonder who they all were and what they were doing up there. Do you suppose that anyone in Smallville USA is wondering that about me?

Look at that! Just over there! The clouds have cut away just a bit like a craggy ledge and I see the sunset still.

The man with his family on the other side of the plane has stood and finally tucked in his shirt to hide his slipping underwear and the crease of his buttocks we have all been forced to see. An excuse to peek into first class and check out the flight attendants' whereabouts. He is sneaking into their loo! The honeymooners, also from the other side, have now occupied the entire row of vacant seats in the middle of the plane. Each to their own end with their blankets, they sleep. It must have been a long reception.

Just picked up Radio Hong Kong on the headsets. Oh no! Japanese disco. "Lorelei." Sorry. I don't think so.

Fast approaching the Northern Star, we shall leave it behind soon. A day, and then the land of the Southern Cross where the sunrise will chase us into Sydney and six months working with Des and Faye Davis at their Theatre in Wollongong, New South Wales. When they suggested this adventure two years ago, it was all I could think about, hope for, save for. Now I was on my way. I had no idea what this new chapter in my life would bring. But I was all too ready for the change. Or so I thought.

*　*　*

Under a rainforest canopy in Kuranda, I walked through the open market not knowing what I was looking for and finding the unexpected. A handmade ocarina fashioned from local clay. A white and flowered sarong made from incredibly soft cotton. And a visit with an insistent fortune teller who called to me from the door of her caravan.

"I'll tell you," she said, quite unsolicited, as though I had asked a question out loud.

"Pardon?" I asked in my fading Canadian accent.

"Come. It's all right," she repeated. "You want to know. I'll tell you. Come. Only sixteen dollars."

Curious now about what my question could possibly have been, I relented.

She had no crystal ball, no tarot cards or incense. No turban or shawl. She was neither young nor old. She was simply a woman inviting me to sit at her table and offer her my hand.

She began. "Your father could be violent."

"What? No, he wasn't," I protested.

"He was not a violent man," she added. "But he could not help what was happening to him, and it caused him to rage at times."

Then I remembered the day Dad threw the jam jar against the dining room wall. What was he angry about? It was the only outburst I had ever seen.

She continued. "The letter A figures greatly in your life. It will have a major impact."

That I could believe. I was going to live in Australia. Once I returned here with my work Visa, I would be running the Young Company for Theatre South and living near the ocean for the rest of my life.

She nodded and then added. "There is someone for you. The one you will be with. He's married but not really. That will pass. He is meant for you."

"Really?" I asked. I couldn't think who she might be talking about. Romance was the farthest thing from my mind. My mind that she seemed to read.

"Not just a romance. You already know each other. You are meant to be together, but you do not know it yet. It's all right. It will come."

That was all she had to tell me. The next day on the last leg of my Queensland holiday, I found my way to Port Douglas where I biked to an empty beach, sat alone wrapped in my sarong and taught myself to play the ocarina. "A" for Australia. I gave no further thought to the rest of her predictions.

*   *   *

It's Saturday night and I'm sitting with Paul and Gail in Jim and Betty's living room. They are all getting a big kick out of my slight Australian accent and having a lot of fun teasing me.

"How was Australia?" Brother Jim wants to know.

"Fantastic! I can't wait to go back."

Betty chimes in. "Mom says you're taking her with you. You are, aren't you?"

"I think so."

"Good. When?"

"Not sure. Whenever I go. I have to get my immigration papers first so I can work down there. But my job starts in about three months, so I'll need them soon."

"So, Freddie, you're going to be an Aussie!" Paul's enthusiasm for my adventure seems quite sincere.

"Did you find your llama rancher? Gonna get married and stay down there forever?" Gail sounds hopeful and who could blame her.

While I was saving for my trip to Australia over the last two years, I'd lived with Paul and Gail and their son, Jason. I was, in fact, now back in their home for the time being. Their generosity may have known no bounds, but it was long past time for me to move on.

"No. I didn't meet a llama rancher. Not many of those in Wollongong. But, yeah, maybe I'll stay down there forever. Give you guys a place to come visit."

Betty needs confirmation.

"And you're taking Mom with you."

"I guess."

"Well, she's already starting to pack, so you better."

Jim changes the subject.

"What are you doing next Sunday?"

"Nothing, I don't think. Why?"

"I've rented the Welland arena for an hour. I thought we'd have a family skate."

"Cool."

"Bring a date."

"A date? I've been gone for six months. Who would I get for a date?"

"Find somebody. It's going to be all couples."

"Great."

Who am I supposed to call, I wondered. I think of the fellows I dated before I left for Australia, but six months is a long time to be away and I'm not comfortable with any of those choices. Maybe I'll ask my old theatre school friend, Doug. He has been touring as Production Manager out of Carousel Players with my Christmas play. He's a good safe choice. That night I give him a call. He agrees.

"Sounds like fun."

He arrived at the arena in dress pants and sweater, ready for a couples' skate, only to be met with a family hockey game. In my defence, I did not know that that was the intention either and wondered if perhaps it was just another family joke on me. But Doug was a good sport and joined in the fun. Later, we all go back to Jim and Betty's for drinks. Sitting in the room with the bar, Paul and Doug are horsing around with motorcycle goggles and everyone is laughing.

And then Betty sits down and the first thing she says to Doug is, "So, when are you going to take her off our hands?"

Some people laugh. Doug doesn't. He doesn't know what to say. I'm mortified. At that moment, I am all too ready to move to another hemisphere.

But in the end, I wasn't sorry to disappoint my family by not moving to Australia. Mom kept asking about the trip, of course. She needed to know the details. When would we go? What should she bring? How much money would she need? She never actually asked how long she could stay with me in Wollongong. Just, when would we go? But as the months rolled past, I began to realize that I may not go back at all.

In the beginning, Doug and I didn't actually date so much as spend time together. Impromptu lunches or visits at the Theatre Centre where we had both been students and he was now on the faculty.

He was always easy to be with. And so I felt comfortable enough to ask if I could hitch a ride to Barrie the next time he went back up to oversee the tour of my play.

"Sure. No problem," he said.

A few days later, as I was finishing up a script meeting in the Carousel rehearsal hall, the stage manager said to me, "Doug is here."

"Who?" I asked, my brain still in writing mode.

"Doug Rathbun. Your ride to Barrie."

"Oh, yeah. Where is he?"

"Sitting in his car waiting for you."

"Oh. Well, I guess I'd better go. Do you want me to leave these changes with you?"

"No, it's okay," the stage manager said. "I got them all."

"Okay. Thanks."

I grabbed the script, my overnight bag and jacket and headed out the back door of the rehearsal hall. Doug was sitting in his black Celica, leaning back and smoking with one knee up on the steering wheel. He was listening to music.

"Hi!" I chirped as I opened the passenger side door.

"Hi!"

He sat up and butted out his cigarette. I tossed my overnight bag into the back seat.

"I didn't know you were here. Why didn't you come in?" I asked.

"I didn't want to interrupt. I figured you'd come out eventually."

"Well, thanks for waiting. And thanks for the lift."

"No problem. I'm going up there anyway. Whereabouts in Barrie are you going?"

"Oh. I have the address. But it's really easy to find. We just need to get off the 400 at Duckworth."

"Duckworth. Sure. I know where that is."

And we were off.

It was a bright November afternoon with plenty of daylight left. We would hit Barrie by five thirty or so and my friends should be home from work by the time we arrived.

"Cigarette?" Doug offered me his pack of John Players Special, already open with two cigarettes pulled part way out for easy access. That was nice.

"Thanks!"

I took a cigarette, and he offered me a light. The first long drag relaxed me, and I settled in.

"So, how was Australia?" he wanted to know.

"Fantastic! I just loved it there. I cannot wait to go back," I said, beaming.

"When are you going back?"

"Well, I don't know, just yet." And I didn't. I explained. "I have the Belle of Amherst tour first. And I have to get my immigration papers, otherwise I can't work there. Des and Faye have offered me a great position in their company."

"How are they?" Doug knows Des and Faye.

"Good! They're good."

We talked with ease about Carousel Players, Des and Faye, the shows we did at Theatre School. We talked about people we both knew, the good friends and the idiots and we had the same opinions of both types. We laughed.

"Cigarette?" He had taken his pack out again.

"Thanks."

We headed north on the 400. The drive was straightforward and easy. Doug leaned back in his seat taking a long drag from his cigarette and steering the car with one knee. Confident. I was not worried at all. Trust. The laughter was good. We had known each other in theatre school, but I didn't recall us ever spending a lot of time together. Still, it seemed as if we had been friends for years. The conversation flowed effortlessly. No pretense. Just comfortable company.

"What time are your friends expecting you?" he wanted to know.

"They're not. I'm going to surprise them. Maybe when we get there I could hop into the trunk of your car. You knock on the door and tell them you have a package for them in your car, and when you open the trunk, I'll jump out!"

"Really? You're going to get into the trunk of my car."

"Sure." My impulsive attitude sustained the logic of my gag. Why not? No worries.

"Oka-ay."

Doug sounded less convinced but was still willing to help.

"I don't know how clean the trunk is."

"Oh, I don't care."

And I didn't. I was wearing jeans and an oversized, faded yellow sweatshirt with the Carousel Players logo emblazoned on the front. But maybe I'd fix my ponytail. I pulled down the visor for the vanity mirror and looked at myself for the first time since I dressed that morning.

"There's a pencil in my head!"

And sure enough, sticking out of the top of my ponytail like a Japanese hair ornament was a bright yellow HB pencil.

"Why didn't you tell me there was a pencil in my head?" I wanted to know.

"I thought you knew," Doug answered.

We laughed. I suppose I should have been embarrassed but I wasn't. The talk continued until we saw the highway sign for the Bracebridge cut off.

"Bracebridge? I think we missed the turnoff," he said. "Which one was it?"

"Duckworth."

I looked back to see if I recognized where we were.

"Yeah, I think we missed it," I said.

"Oh, man. Sorry. How did I miss it? I've driven this highway for years."

Neither one of us had been paying attention to the road. But the mistake didn't matter. He took the ramp, and we doubled back to Barrie.

I missed what should have been our first date, New Years' Eve, because I was never given the message that he had called to ask me out. Be that as it may, a few days later, on January 4 he was good enough to help my brothers finally move me out of Paul and Gail's home. I believe the Universe heard a collective sigh of relief emanating from Welland that day.

I was moving to St. Catharines, where I would be touring with Carousel Players again. I had a long relationship with the company. In the third year of my theatre training, I had apprenticed with Carousel because my major was Theatre For and With Children. And no company did that better than Carousel Players.

For the last thirteen years as a professional actor and playwright I had returned to the company many times performing and touring participation plays and mainstage work. This tour would be different. This would be a one-woman show. *The Belle of Amherst*, by William Luce, was a role I had performed often over the years, in several theatres, including Theatre South in New South Wales. For Carousel, and with the playwright's blessing, I had adapted the work down to a one act play, well suited to the high school market that Carousel was moving into.

My new and temporary home was a two-bedroom apartment on the second floor of an old house, and I'd be sharing it with a couple who were also working with the company that season.

The day of the move my brothers hauled my sofa bed out of Paul and Gail's basement and loaded it onto the rental truck. I was already at the apartment. Doug met us there, much to my brothers' relief, I believe, because for a single person who had been out the country for six months, I had a lot of stuff to move. But the bane of their existence was to be my very heavy, overstuffed, sofa bed. It would serve as the couch in the shared apartment. That was if they could get it up the stairs.

The outdoor stairs were too fragile to attempt. It was a very, very old house. Just inside the front door was the enclosed stairway to the second floor, which Paul, Jim, and Doug eyed suspiciously. This was going to take some engineering expertise because clearly the sofa bed was at least two inches wider than the stairway.

With Paul at one end walking backward and Doug and Jim at the other, the three of them hauled the sofa bed up the front porch steps and set it down. Thud. It was definitely heavy. Picking it up again, they shuffled to the bottom of the indoor stairs. This was do or die time. They were able to squeeze the monstrosity into the dark stairway and move it up one step at a time. Squished against each wall the sofa bed took up all space and it was slow going. At one point Paul accidently let go of his end and fearing the worst he yelled, "Look out!" But nothing happened. Their oversized burden was stuck two feet from the top floor doorway and five inches above the steps. Suspended.

Thinking that it might be best to just take it back down again my brothers suggested that maybe I could do without the mammoth. But it was a moot point since the sofa bed would budge neither up nor down. So now what?

Once they had caught their breaths the three of them agreed that the only thing to do was push it with all their might and hope it ended up in the apartment. Walls and paint be damned. So Paul went down the outside stairs and around the house to join Jim and Doug. Shoulders to the job they counted one, two, three and with all their collective strength, shoved the sofa bed up the last few steps. It flew into the apartment like a blob spurting from a pressurized toothpaste tube and landed with a thud inside the apartment.

Looking down the stairs I saw the three of them, collapsed and gasping in between profanities.

"That thing is never leaving this apartment." Doug panted.

I went to the fridge and got them each a beer.

As it turned out I didn't spend much time in that apartment. Over the next month, Doug and I finally started dating and as we became closer, Australia seemed farther and farther away.

One month from the day that he helped me move, Doug proposed, and I said yes.

It was February 4.

* * *

My feelings had yo-yoed up and down all day. I didn't know what to think anymore.

The move to Calgary, Alberta, had been exciting and adventurous. Exciting because Doug had been recruited by Mount Royal College to design and run the new Technical Theatre Stream for the Department of Fine and Performing Arts. Adventurous because there was no guarantee that the position would become tenure track. Nevertheless, we sold our home and packed up our car. With our one-year-old baby girl, Heather, tucked between the computer and monitor on the back seat, we drove halfway across the country to a new life where we knew absolutely no one. Six weeks later our son, James, was born and for the next nine months life became very busy.

On this particular morning, before Doug left for work, he had told me to start planning our move back east and I nearly cried. Why? Part of me was excited about going to be with family. So I reconciled myself to organizing, believing that the excitement of another adventure would settle my feelings. Then Doug called to say that they think he may be offered a twelve-month contract. Now what the hell did that mean? Was it worth staying for? Could we risk it? Were we staying? Should I call a realtor or not?

Then Mom called. I had to tell her. She was planning her summer trip west. But how best to approach the subject? Gingerly.

So, I asked her, "Can you get a refund on your flight?"

"Why?" she wanted to know.

"We may be coming home."

"To stay?"

"Yes."

"Oh."

There is an interminable silence. And then, "No, I can't get a refund."

I could see her face sinking in disappointment. Her initial shock had to do with her losing her trip west. It didn't seem to sink in what was happening to us, to me. I tried to comfort her by saying, "I'm sure you can get a refund if you cancel within twenty-one days."

And then the predictable conversation begins.

Mom sighs. "I'll have to go down there and see what I can do."

"Don't go. Call."

"What will I do?"

How I hated this feigned helplessness.

"Call," I tell her. "Call and ask if you can get a refund within twenty-one days."

"What do I ask?"

What is wrong with this picture, I think to myself. I'm the one in turmoil here. Suddenly, that small part of me that was anxious to go back remembered all the catering and coddling and dealing with. Suddenly, I was exhausted. But she persists.

"I'll have to go down there."

"Just call!" I snap at her, and it seems to change her tone.

"No, no. I have to go down there anyway."

So, it's not a problem after all. She's just trying to make me feel guilty. I can't stand this.

"Sorry I loused up your holiday. I shouldn't have told you."

Then, there it was again. That involuntary ache that warned of the forthcoming tears which had plagued me for days now. She must have heard it in my voice because now she turned motherly and comforting.

"It's all right, Poodie. What's happening?"

"They haven't offered Doug anything yet, but we think it may be another short contract. We can't afford it."

"So, you'll be coming home?"

Has the penny finally dropped for her? Is she perhaps happy about that possible outcome? I wonder.

"Well, won't it be nice to have us home. Isn't that better than a holiday?"

"Yes, dear. Oh, and Jayne will be thrilled. She's missed you so. No, no. Please don't worry about the money."

And then she tops it off with one more dig.

"Oh, all my beautiful clothes I bought for the trip! Oh, well."

"I'm sorry!" No hiding it now. I'm crying.

"Don't be upset. Winn, are you upset? Everything is going to be all right, dear. Don't you know what the Bible says?"

"What?" I know what's coming.

"All things work out for the best. And you come under my umbrella."

I guess that means God will be good to me because I'm good to her. I know that's what it means. It's the way most of my life's achievements have been credited. But that is not why I'm crying. I just want to know what the hell the decision is, and I don't want to have to worry about disappointing my poor, disappointed mother anymore.

*　　*　　*

Mom has been visiting us in Calgary for more than a week now. And although we suggested that a ten-day stay would be lovely, she is here for at least another week. Her second visit this year. Her fifth since Doug became tenured faculty at Mount Royal. She has been sitting at the kitchen table reading the newspaper while I finish up the dishes. It's been a busy morning.

"Can we go out for lunch? My treat."

"Sure, Mom. Where would you like to go?"

"Well, I don't know. What's around?"

"There's a Gramma Lee's across the street in the mall. They make great sandwiches."

"Will the children eat there?"

"Sure. They can share a sandwich. Or I can feed them first and just buy them a drink."

"Oh, good. Let's do that."

"Okay. Heather! James!" I call up the stairs. "Come and get a sandwich. We're going over to the mall with Gramma."

"I am hungry," Mom says.

"Yes, Mom. It will just take me a few minutes to get the kids ready. I need to feed them first."

"Don't worry about me. I'll just wait here. Is there any tea left?"

"Tea? Maybe. But it will be cold."

"Oh, dear. I can't stand cold tea. I'll put the kettle on."

She gets up and walks over to the stove.

Heather comes into the kitchen and I ask her, "Where's your brother?"

"Upstairs, Mommy."

"James, come on down and get a sandwich."

Then I look over at Mom leaning against the stove watching my teapot begin to heat up. "Mom! That's not the kettle!"

"I just thought I'd warm up the teapot on the stove."

"You can't put that teapot on a burner, Mom. It's pottery."

"Oh. Well, I don't know."

"Here, I'll put the kettle on for you. You just sit down."

"Oh, don't worry about me." She answers, making her way back to the table. "I can make a cup of tea, for heaven's sake."

I put the kettle on while Heather and James come into the kitchen.

"Mommy, can I have peanut butter and jelly?" Heather asks.

"Yes, dear. James, do you want peanut butter and jelly too?"

"Yes."

"Okay. Two peanut butter and jelly sandwiches. Milk for you, Heather?"

"Yes, please, Mommy. And apple juice for James."

"Okay. Sit at the table with Gramma."

James tries to pull himself up onto a chair but can't quite manage it so Heather pushes him up.

"No! I can do it myself!" he protests.

"James, your sister is just trying to help."

"I do it myself." And he does.

"Here's your milk and your juice."

"Winn, the kettle is boiling."

"Yes, Mom, I know. I'll get it."

"I hope you have sugar. I can do without milk, but I can't bear tea without sugar."

"Still have sugar. Had sugar this morning."

"Where is it?" Mom looks around the table.

"Here. It's right here."

"Oh, good. Do you have a spoon?"

"Here."

"Winn, the kettle is boiling."

"I know."

"Mommy, can I have more apple juice?" James asks.

Mom corrects him. "May I?"

"What?"

She corrects him again. "Pardon me."

"Gramma means you should say, *May* I have more juice."

"And don't say 'what.' Why doesn't he say 'pardon me'?"

"Oh, I don't know." Then to myself I mutter, "Maybe because he's two?"

"Is the tea ready yet?"

"Coming. James, here's your juice, Sweetie."

"Thank you," he says, taking the glass in both hands.

"Aw. That's better." She approves.

"Here we are. Two peanut butter and jelly sandwiches and a cup of tea."

I place everything on the table.

"Is there milk?" she asks.

"Yes. Here you are."

She pours a huge amount of milk into her mug while gazing out the kitchen bay window. The kids eat in silence. I sit.

"Good sandwich, Mommy." Heather says as she and James finish their lunch.

"Thank you, Sweetie. Are you full?"

"Yes. Let's go!"

"Okay. Just as soon as Gramma finishes her tea."

"Oh, you don't need to wait on me," Mom says, pushing her teacup aside. "Let's go."

"But your tea?"

"Ach! Stone cold."

"Okay. Come on, guys." I say to my children.

"Gramma too?"

"Yes, Heather. Gramma too."

"Don't worry about me. Go on down the stairs. I'll be right behind."

I turn on the answering machine, grab my purse and head to the stairs that lead down to the front door of our townhouse.

"Take my hand down the stairs, James."

"No. I can do it myself." And he does.

"Shoes, everybody."

She is coming down the stairs one step at a time, but I can't stop to watch and make sure.

"Heather, Honey, get the door so I can get the stroller out."

"Okay."

"Thanks."

Shoes on, jackets zipped, stroller out onto the driveway, wheels locked.

Heather in first . . .

"Oh dear." Mom watches. "Do we have to wait to do all that?"

"They need to go in the stroller, Mom."

"Oh, dear."

She sits down on the front porch wicker chair.

"Okay, Heather. In you go. Come on James."

Mom sighs. "Are you nearly ready?"

"Yes, Mom. I just need to lock the door."

"I think I'll just go up to the bathroom one more time before we leave."

She heads back into the house and up the stairs.

"Where's Gramma going?" Heather asks me.

"She'll be right back."

But she's not. Eventually, the kids begin to fuss.

"Heather, don't!" James complains.

"What's going on?"

"I just hugged him," Heather says.

"I said don't!" James shrugs away from his sister and begins to stand in the stroller.

"What are you doing, James? Sit back down."

"I don't want her to hug me."

"Well, if you sit in front of her, she's going to hug. Do you want to walk?"

"No."

"Do you want to sit behind?"

"No."

"Then sit back down."

He starts to cry.

"Oh, dear. What is wrong with him? Is he teething?" Mom has reappeared.

"Yes. But mostly he's restless. They both are."

"Well, let's go, for heaven's sake."

"Okay. I'll just lock the door. And we're off!"

"You left the milk on the table."

"Oh. You put it away?"

"No. I don't where you keep it."

"Just in the fridge," I say.

"Let's go. I'm dying for a cup of tea."

The day is sunny, and the walk is short. She lags behind, four paces as always. As the kids and I reach the corner lights I stop and wait.

"Mommy, the sign says Walk." Heather says.

"I know, Honey. We'll just wait for Gramma."

"Don't wait for me. I'm coming," Mom calls.

We wait anyway.

The doors to the mall are manual so as I let her walk ahead of us, I ask "Mom, can you get the door?"

"Oh, sure."

She steps in front of me, opens the door, goes into the mall, and the door closes behind her. O –kay. I turn the stroller around and push the door open with my butt.

"There you are." She has turned to see me with the kids in the stroller. "Where is this restaurant?"

"Right there, Mom. Gramma Lee's."

"Oh. It's a cafeteria."

"Sort of, yes."

"I didn't think it was a cafeteria."

Gramma Lee's is right on the first corner inside the mall and there are no walls which makes it easy to park the stroller next to an outside table. Mom sits.

"Okay, James, up you come. You sit here. Come on Heather, Honey, you're next."

I sit.

"What do they serve?" Mom wants to know.

"Mostly soup and sandwiches."

"Oh, no. It's too hot for soup. What are you going to have?"

"Well, they make a great chicken salad sandwich. It's actually my favourite."

"No. What else do they have?"

"Pretty much everything. Roast beef, turkey, tuna, cheese, ham . . ."

"Ham?"

"Yes. Do you want a ham and cheese sandwich?"

"No. I don't eat pork."

"What do you eat?"

"Anything. I'm not fussy."

"What about a roast beef sandwich?"

"No. What are you having?"

"I'm going to have chicken salad."

"No, I don't want chicken salad. What else do they have?"

"How about turkey or tuna?"

"I can have tuna at home."

"Mommy, can I have a cookie?" Heather wants to know.

"I think so, Honey." I stand.

"Where are you going?" Mom sounds a little panicked.

"I have to go up to the counter to order. They make the sandwiches fresh."

"So, it's a cafeteria?"

"Sort of."

"Here."

She presses a ten-dollar bill into my hand.

"Is that enough?" She wants to know.

"I think so. Depends on what you want."

"I don't want a lot. Maybe we can share a sandwich."

"Sure. What kind?"

"What kind do you want?"

"I want chicken salad."

"Oh, no. I don't like chicken salad. But you go ahead."

"What do you like?" I ask again.

"Anything. I'm not fussy."

"Anything but ham?"

"I don't eat pork. It's unclean."

"It's ham," I say.

"Just get me whatever you think is good."

"Roast beef?"

"No, I don't think so."

"Cheese?"

"What kind of cheese?"

"Probably cheddar."

"Hmmm."

She rests her elbow on the table and her face in her hand.

"I'll just get you a roast beef sandwich. Okay? Alberta beef. You'll like it."

"Whatever you think, dear. I'm not fussy."

I leave her at the table with my two small children and head over to the sandwich counter. One roast beef on brown with mustard, one chicken salad on brown with lettuce, two juice drink boxes, two chocolate chip cookies, one iced tea, and one pot of hot tea. Pay, pick up the tray, and head back to the table with our lunch.

"Mom! Where are the kids?"

She's alone at the table!

"Hmmm?"

"Heather and James! Where are the kids?"

"Oh. I think they went down the mall."

"What? Why?" I plop the tray down onto the table spilling some of her tea.

171

"I don't know. They wanted to."

"And you let them?"

"What could I do?"

She does that crying thing with her voice.

"Mom! They're two and three years old! God! Which way did they go?"

Panic. It's a small mall but a mall, nonetheless. I don't wait for her to answer. Out of the restaurant, past the grocery store, the bank, the post office, the bakery, the other bank, and a clear view of the other end of the mall. There they are, looking in the window of the pet shop. I slow my steps as I get nearer.

"What are you two doing here?"

"James wanted to see the puppies," Heather answers.

"You know you're not supposed go off on your own. Why didn't you stay with Gramma?"

"I had to stay with James."

"Come on. Come back and have your cookies."

With James on my hip and Heather's hand in mine we head back to Gramma Lee's.

"Well, there you are." Mom says to me.

"They were at the pet shop. Come on, guys. Sit down and have your cookies."

I sit. She pours her tea then picks up her sandwich.

"What kind of sandwich is this?"

"Roast beef, Mom. I think you'll like it."

Her first bite seems to confirm that it's a good sandwich, and she pours her tea.

"What time is Doug home from work?"

"Today? Probably about five. His last class ends at four. There's no rehearsal today." Finally, a bite of my sandwich.

"What will you make for dinner?"

"Not sure. Pork chops. No. Maybe meatloaf and mash. How is your sandwich?"

"It's all right. That looks good. What have you got?"

"Chicken salad."

"Hmmm. Maybe I should have had that."

She takes a large gulp of her tea, then puts the cup down in disappointment. "Ach. Stone cold."

*　　*　　*

"Mommy please! I hate the white! I just hate it! Can't I just have some colour?"

I stopped in mid action and looked down at Heather from the oak chair where I stood putting the finishing touches of clouds across the top of the walls. I thought the painting project was going well. Heather had had so much fun sponging the warm colours on her own bedroom walls. She even seemed to take pride in covering all evidence of artwork from earlier years—magic marker sketches and scribbles from long ago temper tantrums and fits of clarification. Her long, neat braid lay down the back of her tie dye shirt. On a chair of her own she had worked contentedly on the closet doors, sponging stars in assorted colours and hand painting the crescent moon with her own water colour brush. Singing along to her Fred Penner cassette she had given no indication that the room was not shaping up exactly the way she wanted it to. No indication at all. And now that we were nearly done, and I had perfected my cloud painting technique she was saying she didn't like it.

"But these are clouds, Heather. They're part of your skyscape."

"Mommy! They're white! I hate white."

"White is beautiful and clean. What's wrong with it? I worked hard to make this room nice for you, and you stand there and tell me you don't like it? Anyway, the walls are mostly lilac."

"But then you put on the white. It's my room. Can't you please get rid of the white?'

"White is nice."

173

"But Mommy, I hate it. You make EVERYTHING white."

"No, I don't." I was too tired for this. We were both too hot and tired. Then the words flew out of my mouth before I could stop them, as if they had a will of their own. "How dare you speak to me that way! Who do you think you are? Shame on you!"

I gasped when I heard what I had said. Shame on you? Shame? Oh, God, I thought. I sound just like my mother. Please, God, don't let this day be a lasting, traumatic memory in my daughter's life. Fix it. Fix it! Say something fair and enlightened to her, quickly, before she feels shame of any kind.

"Oh, Heather, I'm sorry. Don't cry. Don't cry, Honey. Come here. I'm sorry." I pulled her to me and held her close.

"Do I really make everything white?"

"Yes." She wiped the tears from her face with both hands, still defiant in her opinion.

Then I looked around the room. My god. She was right. White clouds, bed, toy box, duvet. Look at it. Clean, pure white. Not much doubt about what I'm compensating for. This had to stop.

"Oh, honey. I'm sorry. Don't cry. You know what?"

"What?"

"You're right. A lot of the room is white."

"I hate it. It's boring."

"Okay. Fair enough. Let's get a cold drink and cool down. And if it's not too late by then, we'll fix the paint the way you want it. Okay?"

"Kay."

"We'll go over to the Seven Eleven and get a cold drink."

"A Slurpee?"

"Sure. How about a red pop Slurpee?"

"Yeah. Red pop."

Heather tossed her braid back behind her shoulder, her tear-streaked face now beaming in expectation.

"Mommy, why do they call it red pop?"

"Because it's red. It's really cream soda."

"*Cream* soda?"

"Yes. But Aunt Jayne and I always called it red pop."

"They had red pop when you were little?"

"Yes."

"Wow."

Wow. How could there ever have been a time when your parents were seven years old and drank red pop?

* * *

Mom is visiting again. We're sitting at the kitchen table, talking. Doug is at work, but summer vacation has begun for our kids so I'm trying to think of things for us to do.

"How far away is Lethbridge?" she asks.

"About an hour and a half. Why?"

"I suppose it has changed a lot since we lived there."

"You lived in Lethbridge? When?"

"Well, we didn't live *in* Lethbridge. We lived on a ranch. My dad got a job as a kind of foreman. And Mother was in charge of the meals. For the ranch hands."

"Why did you move to Lethbridge?"

"It was Dad's idea. This all happened, oh, it would have been the late 20s. During the Depression. I was only ten or so. Thousands of people were out of work. There was no work for Dad in Bathurst. So, we took one of the government's special trains from the east coast to the west to help with the harvest."

"I never knew that. Did you want to go back? I could keep the car one day."

"No."

"Are you sure? We could make it a day trip."

"No. I have no desire to go to Lethbridge."

"But maybe we could find the ranch."

"Oh, I don't know. I don't remember where it was."

She pauses for a moment, thinking.

"I do remember there was a Chinese cook there who still had his que or pigtail. That fascinated me. The ranch was owned by two Hindu gentlemen from India. They couldn't go home again because one of them had cut his hair, but the other still wore a turban. We only lived there a short time."

"Just for harvest?" I ask.

But she answers, "How I loved that ranch. The Rockies within sight. The magnificent sunsets."

She sits now, elbows on the table and folded hands against her cheek. She's gazing out our kitchen window remembering something I cannot see. Where does she go? I leave her at the table and begin to stack the dishwasher.

"Jim," Mother said. "Pull down the upper berth and lay out our mattress. I am going to heat up our tea before someone else takes over the stove."

What a long, weary trip. Bathurst to Montreal to Toronto. Then all through Northern Ontario. The scenery had been spectacular, and Cathy loved it. The rail line cut through hundreds of miles of forest and rock. Each bend in the journey presented another vista of lakes and blazes of late summer colour where trees were just beginning to turn. How many days ago was that?

Their tea that night was a slice of smoked lamb, which Mother reheated on the stove and served with two biscuits each and a slice of cheese. And of course, hot, sweet tea to drink. Afterward, as usual, Father slept in the seat below the bunk that Cathy shared with Mother. Another night and they would awaken in windy Winnipeg. Then Winnipeg to Lethbridge where they transferred to a milk train, much to Mother's dismay, until they finally disembarked somewhere outside of the city.

"What a relief." Mother sighed.

"Wait here with the luggage." Father said, leading them to a bench outside the small station. "I'll go check on our transportation to the ranch."

"Another train?" Cathy asked.

Father smiled, "I don't think so. Just stay with your mother." And he disappeared into the building. But Mother did not sit. She paced back and forth in front of the bench, walking off her apprehension, while the locomotive idled and hissed as though calling them back on board.

Finally, she saw her husband as he came around the corner of the station.

"Jim, there you are." she said.

"Right," he answered. "Cathy, help your mother with the luggage. I'll take the trunk. This way."

They followed him through the station house and out the other side where their ride to the ranch was waiting.

It was an open, flat, buckboard wagon sitting high on four large wooden wheels. It had two leather bench seats, one behind the other and was hitched to two horses, one grey, one white.

"Horses!" Cathy gasped.

She immediately fell in love with the animals. They were different from the horses she remembered back home in Perth where, as a little girl, she had learned to ride side saddle, trotting along the river Tey and through the parks with Grandad. But they were horses, nonetheless. "Hello," she whispered. The grey horse bobbed its head toward her and gave a slight neigh. Cathy laughed.

"Nice to meet you, too." she said to the horse.

"Cathy. Come away from that animal." Mother's stern voice cut through the welcome.

"Yes, Mother."

Then whispering to the horse, she said, "See you later."

The tall and rumpled ranch hand who had hopped down from the buckboard now helped Cathy and her mother up onto the back bench while Father and another fellow loaded their luggage and trunk onto a second horse and wagon. Then he climbed up onto the front seat of the buckboard and they set off on the last leg of the journey.

"Mom?" I ask again as I sit back down at the table.

"Hmm?" Her gaze returns from the horizon.

"I said did you ever see a steam-powered threshing machine?"

"Oh, sure. I was allowed to drive the horses—four of them, on the threshing machine," she says quite matter of factly.

"You were? You mean you worked in the fields, not the kitchen with your mother and the cook?"

"Well, I spent a lot of time in the big kitchen of the ranch, too. The old time Five Roses Cookbook, I remember. The meals were tremendous because the men worked very hard in the fields. But Five Roses Cookbook or not, once I learned how to ride Western style, I was a better cowboy than a cook. Is there any more tea?"

"Sure," I say. "I'll put the kettle back on."

"Oh, don't bother if it's not made."

"It's okay. It will only take a few minutes."

"Well, I think I'll just lie down for a bit until it's ready."

"Sure. It won't be long."

She gets up from the table and walks upstairs to lie down on her bed. Heather and James are watching the Sharon, Lois, and Bram TV show in the living room. I rinse out our teacups and put the kettle back on to boil. I know she will probably doze off to sleep again and the pot will go cold. But that really doesn't matter anymore. Upstairs, Mom closes her eyes.

"There is nothing more magnificent than a western sky when the sun sets behind the Rockies" Cathy thinks. How she loves it here. She has gone out the back kitchen door to take a long walk in the evening air, beyond the corral and leaving the ranch house far in the distance.

Behind her, one of the horses neighs and she turns to walk back and visit them. Then she sees the grey mare bolt out of the corral. Another horse follows. Now one of the ranch hands hollers, "Look out! Look out!" Someone has neglected to shut the corral gate. All but one of the ranch hands are on foot and running toward her but too far away to stop the escape. Five horses now, clear the gate and make for the open field. Without thinking, Cathy runs after them, waving her arms and yelling, "Haw! Haw! Haw!" like she has heard the wranglers call. She makes a wide circle and comes out in front of them, still yelling. At the front of the pack, the grey horse slows up and turns, slowing to a trot to pass her. "Haw! Haw!" she hollers. Now three ranch hands appear behind her and take up the call. Together with the one on horseback they round up all the horses and maneuver them back to the corral.

"I remember. I was taken home by one of the cowboys, riding before him on his horse. I was the heroine of the night. Could have been trampled."

"Mom? Are you awake?"

"Better cowboy than a cook," she murmurs.
"Mom? Are you dreaming?"
She opens her eyes and looks at me. "Oh. Is the tea ready?"
"No. But I can make another pot."
"Oh, don't bother. What time is dinner?"
"As soon as Doug gets home."
"I suppose I can wait until then."

That is the end of the Lethbridge conversation. But I can't help trying to imagine my mother as a cowboy.

* * *

"Hello?"

"Poodie, am I losing my mind?"

"Mom? What's the matter?"

"Betty said my mind is going and I'll have to move out of my apartment."

She's crying on the phone.

"What? Why would she do that?"

"Am I losing my mind?"

"Oh Mom, don't listen to Betty."

"That's what Paul said."

"Then just listen to him and never mind what Betty says. She only upsets you."

"Do you think so?"

"Yes."

"You would tell me, wouldn't you, if I was losing my mind?"

"Yes."

She may be forgetful, sure. She's eighty. But she is not insane.

"You're not losing your mind, Mom."

"Oh, thank you. I feel so much better now."

A few minutes of small talk and she hangs up. What the hell is wrong with Betty, to say such a thing to Mom? Then one minute later the phone rings again.

"Hello?"

"Poodie, am I losing my mind?"

"Mom?"

"Betty said my mind is going and I'll have to move out of my apartment. Am I losing my mind?"

"I told you, don't listen to Betty."

"You did?"

"Yes."

"You would tell me, wouldn't you, if I was losing my mind?"

"You're not, Mom. You're fine."

"Oh, thank you. I feel so much better now."

"Okay, Mom. Just try to relax."

She hangs up. That was odd. Even for Mom. One minute later the phone rings again.

"Hello?"

"Poodie, am I losing my mind?"

"Mom?"

"Betty said my mind is going and I'll have to move out of my apartment. Am I losing my mind?"

"I told you, don't listen to Betty."

"You did?"

"Yes."

"When?" she asks.

"We just had this exact conversation."

"We did?"

"Yes. You've just called me three times and said exactly the same thing."

Now her voice does that fearful, crying thing but this time I believe it is truly justified.

"Oh no! Don't tell me that! I don't remember doing that! I am. I'm losing my mind. Oh, dear God!"

Why did I say that to her? I shouldn't have said that to her. But I don't know what's going on in Ontario. I only know that my mother has called me three times in a row. She's rewinding her fear over and over again.

"I'm sorry Mom. I'm sorry. It's okay. Please don't cry."

"Did I really just call you?"

"It's okay."

"How can it be okay! Oh, dear God."

"Mom, please. Just don't talk to Betty."

"That's what Paul said. That I should not listen to Betty."

"Then just trust Paul. Okay? He'll do what's right for you."

"Yes. Yes, I suppose so."

"Of course. Are you okay?"

"Yes. I'll be fine. Don't worry about me. Just trust Paul, you say."

"Yes, Mom. Trust Paul."

"All right. That's what I'll do then. That's what I'll do. And I'm not losing my mind?"

"No Mom. You're okay."

But now I'm the one who is frightened.

PART FOUR

WALTZ OF LIFE

Jayne's fingers were black with newsprint. Oh great. It wasn't the scrubbing of her hands she would resent so much as the inevitable eczema attack that would follow. The floor was covered now in crumpled bits of old news, broken cardboard boxes and ragged photos, each one wrinkled, torn or imprinted with indelible tea stains. Stains. Those were the prevalent things here. Everything was stained, torn, chipped, or broken. Remnants of the old.

"Oh God." murmured Gail as she gingerly dropped the wrapping of a cracked and dirty dinner plate.

"How old do you think this egg is?"

"Who knows?"

Jayne had long since gotten over her hatred of eggs. She had learned at sixteen how good they could taste when cooked in your own home. She knew, too, that they did not need to be runny or rubbery and that in most homes, eggs were not cooked until black around the edges. And peas were more than shells and chicken wasn't supposed to be pink in the middle. Poor Mom. She never did learn to cook.

Jayne remembered how Winn once told her she thought Mom may have poisoned herself with bad food for so long that her mind finally went. Maybe it was the dirty cast iron frying pan or the aluminum cookware. They were saying now that there seemed to be a connection between aluminum and Alzheimer's, weren't they? Any excuse. Winn was always looking for an excuse for Mom. And why not? As far as Mom was concerned there was only Winn. Winn's education. Winn's acting career. Winn's playwrighting career. Winn's bloody perfect life! Well, it wasn't lovely Winn sitting here digging through this crap, was it?

"What about Winn? What did she say she wanted?"

Gail had an uncanny knack of picking up other peoples' thoughts whether she knew it or not.

"Her Punkinhead mug."

"Her what?"

"The mug she drank out of when she was a little girl. Did you see it when you packed?"

"What the hell is a Punkinhead?"

"Never mind. I'll know it when I see it. Want another beer?"

"Sure."

Jayne high stepped over the newspaper and opened the fridge. She grabbed two long necked bottles of Labatt's Blue and closed the door with her foot. Twisting the cap off the first bottle hurt. Her hands were already starting to feel cracked and dry. Well, she could still open a beer. She handed the open bottle to Gail and twisted the top off her own.

"Thanks. We should just throw it all out, you know." That was Gail's opinion. Gentle Gail, the long-suffering daughter-in-law. "It's all garbage as far as I can see."

Which was why Jayne was there. There had to be something here that only Kay Bray's children would recognize as being of value. Some bit of something. And it was important to try and get it done before Paul came home from work. God knows, he'd had enough of this mess, and it wasn't over yet. Not by a long shot. He and Gail had spent months arranging doctor appointments and psychologist assessments to say nothing of the bureaucratic red tape that threatened to strangle their own sanity as they worked to move Mom into Sunset Haven, Home for the Aged. Paul did not need to see his mother's life divided into garbage worth keeping and garbage worth chucking.

"I don't see anything that looks like the jewelry box Karen wanted."

"Me either," Gail sighed, somewhat unconcerned.

Karen had gone to visit her grandmother in the hospital while she was there for observation, and she called Paul frequently to get updates. She had asked for some box that Mom had promised her years ago.

"It's probably gone," Gail's answered. "Gramma just gave stuff away, you know. Who knows who got it? Some church friend, probably."

Gail always called Mom "Gramma. Gramma Bray." But she was the only adult who ever got away with it.

"Look. Wedgewood," Jayne said, holding the gentle item.

The small blue dish had been wrapped with care in glossy magazine paper. No smear of newsprint. No chips.

"Yeah. Paul and I gave her that a long time ago. There was a teacup and saucer too, but it's gone."

"You'd better keep it, Gail."

"Thanks."

"That's it for this box."

Jayne grabbed the edge of the orange crate with one hand and started scooping crumpled newspaper with the other.

"There's nothing in this, is there?" She gave the large wad of paper a shake.

"Nope."

Gail tilted her pilsner glass and poured the golden beer with skill. Just a quarter inch head was all you wanted on a beer. Then, with a gentle thud, something hit the floor.

"Except for that."

For a silent moment, they looked at each other.

"What is it?" Gail asked.

Jayne cocked her head sideways then bent down to examine the prize.

"It's a cat."

"A what?"

"A cat. A saltshaker shaped like a cat. You want it?"

"Yeah right." Gail sipped her perfect beer. "Where's the pepper?"

"No pepper. Just salt."

"Pass. Maybe Karen wants it."

Jayne set the shaker on the table and wiped her hands on her jeans. God. Everything was so greasy. Years and years of greasy. What a job. Another box to open.

Then she saw it. She recognized it immediately. There was no mistaking the colour, the shape. There was only one of these in all the world.

"Gail, why did you pack this?"

She lifted the basin out of the box.

"I packed everything." Gail looked up from her task long enough to light a Du Maurier.

"I didn't want to try and sort it all myself. Why? What is it?"

"It's the basin."

"The what?"

Jayne lifted the offensive object with her finger and thumb and held it away from her body.

"The basin. The old, putrid coloured sink, wash-dishes, soak-feet, stick-by-the-couch to-throw-up-in-when-sick basin."

"Yuck. Sorry."

"No, no. I'm glad. So glad."

"You want it?"

"Oh yes."

Jayne stepped over the boxes and ceremoniously set the basin upside down on a clear space of the floor.

"Jesus. What do you want that for?" Gail asked.

"For this."

Feet together and with determined accuracy Jayne jumped and came down full force on the back of the basin, buckling it in the middle.

"And this!"

Another jump and crush. Then, with a flood of fury, long bottled and pressurized, she jumped and stomped and ground the basin into a grotesque twist of plastic.

"This! This! This! Fucking basin!"

Gail sat dumbfounded. And when there was nothing left to crush, Jayne kicked the twisted wreckage down the cellar stairs, wiped her hand together in victory and sat back down at the kitchen table.

"Boy that felt good. I knew there had to be something of value in all this stuff."

Gail put her cigarette down into the amber ashtray and covered her mouth with both slender hands as though they weren't wide enough on their own to contain her laughter. The giggle that had been building inside her burst out in a loud, uncharacteristic guffaw. Jayne threw back her head howled out loud.

It was quite uncontrollable now. Quite beyond hope. The echo of sense in her head told Jayne that none of this was funny, but she couldn't stop. It had become too absurd. The flood gates flew open. Snorting, punch drunk, gasping hoots. Tears began to well up in Gail's eyes.

"Stop it, Jayne! Stop it!" Gail pleaded as she crossed her legs and struggled to sit at the table. "Ow, ow. Oh God, that's awful."

"I know."

Breathe. Try to control yourself.

"I know. But I don't know why."

Jayne wiped the tears from her eyes and sighed.

"I don't know why."

The laugher felt good. Warm and fluid. Healing. In her mind's eye she could see the wound, some small festering wound within her, wash over with the laughter and begin to close. She would heal. One cut at a time, she would heal.

Gail got up and pulled a Kleenex from the tissue box on her kitchen counter then plopped back down into the wooded chair, still holding her aching belly.

"I think we're going a little nuts," she said.

"Yeah. Me too. But who wouldn't?"

Jayne picked up her beer and took a good long swig.

"God. That felt good."

Then with a sly look sideways at her sister-in-law she ventured,

"So, you don't want the cat?"

"Gimme that!"

Gail grabbed the offending saltshaker and dropped it into the box designated for garbage. "This is the box that's going to fill up first."

Back to work. A margarine container. Garbage. One stained cloth table napkin. Garbage. A book. Gramma Bray was always buying books at garage sales and flea markets. Famous titles and anything more than fifty years old. Gail doubted that they were ever read, but it made Gramma Bray feel good to have classics on the shelf. Better check the book. Yesterday, Paul had found a total of fifty-three dollars stashed within the covers of six different such books. She held *The Good Earth* by its once loved fragile cover and shook it. Nothing. Pile it with the others. Another chipped mug. Another cracked saucer. One pickle dish with three molded sections. That may be of use. But the rest was garbage.

"Wait!" Jayne's shout made Gail jump.

"Geez! What?"

"That's it! The blue mug."

"This thing? It's no good. Look at it. There's a crack all the way around it. You couldn't use this again."

"I know," Jayne said, still staring at the mug. "But it's Winn's. It's her Punkinhead mug."

"You're kidding. This is what she wants? Good thing you were here 'cause I would have just thrown it out."

"Yeah. Good thing."

Jayne took the mug in both sore hands. She hadn't seen it in years. But the familiarity of it was unmistakeable. It conjured images of snow forts, toboggans, and tinsel. Tall Christmas trees and the Santa Claus parade. There had been a life before the cold-water flat when they lived in their big house on the edge of the city, one step from the river, two streets from Cullimore's farm.

Dance of the Sugar Plum Faeries was baked within the porous crevices of the mug. Their childhood. Angels in the snow. Sleeping back-to-back in their four-poster bed. The house, the yard, the stubble of Dad's beard. The smell of his tobacco, his Old Spice. The soft cold fur of Mom's muskrat coat and Christmas cards with sparkling snow. There had been a time before—before, when Dad was well, and Mom was happy.

Suddenly, she knew why Winn had wanted it, this cool blue, broken mug. It now seemed the most precious thing of all. Maybe it had always been cracked. It didn't matter. It was perfection. It remembered the warmth long gone, the laughter nearly forgotten, and the reasons people forgive.

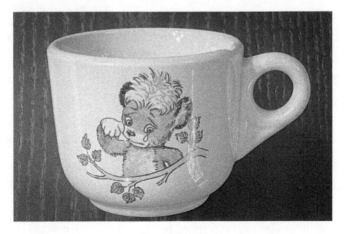

Punkinhead

* * *

I first saw my sister's hat on a hot, humid, punishing summer's day in Ontario. A summer when we had gathered our family of four and made the biennial trek east from Calgary to Ontario, the place of all our births save James. Our sweet Baby James had come into the world to complete our small family just six weeks after our relocation to the West and was therefore the only true Calgarian among us.

Distance from our family was a heavy price to pay for our relocation, but we kept ties as strong as possible with phone calls, letters, Christmas packages that crossed the Prairies in both directions, family trips to visit us in the west and, yes, biennial trips east, sometimes by plane but more often than not via the Trans-Canada road trip.

Two weeks in Ontario would see us housed in a number of locations as our relatives shared the generosity of their homes with us. Doug's parents in St. Catharines, Paul and Gail in Welland, Jayne in Hamilton, and Paul and Nancy in Ridgeville. Everyone got their share of us at one time or another. But wherever we stayed, our families always tried to bring us all together from time to time. In my naiveté, I had always pictured such gatherings as being the norm for our families, especially the siblings who lived near each other. In our own distant western home that boasted no blood relatives but the four of us, I just assumed that everyone in Ontario saw each other regularly. I envisioned joyful Christmas parties and summer barbecues. And while this was sometimes the case, I was to learn that more often than not, it was the exception rather than the rule. So, the arrival and parcelling out of accommodation for the four of us provided an opportunity to get together. One such opportunity was the Burlington Jazz Festival at which our sister, Jayne, had been invited to sing.

It was an outdoor venue, a small stage backing onto Burlington Bay. It was also the perfect stage for Jayne to share with her family her great passion and rare talent, her incredible voice. We piled into our respective vehicles and headed out to Hamilton to pick up Jayne and her youngest son.

On that hot, humid, blistering summer day in Ontario our sister took centre stage. She was amazing. She was confident, animated, totally engaged in her music, and, of course, pitch perfect. Three numbers. It's possible that she sang Hoagie Carmichael and Sarah Vaughan. But what I most clearly remember is her rendition of "Over the Rainbow." She began traditionally, gently, predictably as one would hope to begin life. But neither Jayne nor her life were any of these things.

Once her audience was comfortable with what they thought was to follow, Jayne opened her attitude wide and let loose a raw part of her soul. A full-blown challenge to the Universe. "IF BIRDS FLY OVER THE RAINBOW, THEN WHY! WHY CAN'T I?" [2]She was angry, challenging. She was pissed as only Jayne could be.

Wow. Some of her audience, perhaps even some of her family, wondered what had just happened. Others were hit full force with the power of her voice and passion. But no one could deny the courage of her choice. This was a direct demand for a life she deserved but feared in her heart she may never have. And she used this, the first of many stages to come, to tell the world.

Then her gig was over. Her performance done, Jayne exited stage left and came down the steps to greet her family. Hugging first her son, she met the rest of us beside the seating area, still aglow with the aftermath of performance and all the residual energy that live music creates.

"So, what did you think?" She was smiling.

How did we greet her, we her family, who should have been her greatest fans? Some of us gushed, some were homogenous in praise, and some were non-committal and even embarrassed by her lack of

---

2.   Somewhere Over the Rainbow, Harold Arlen, 1939

convention. But for all of us it was memorable. For me it is memorable to this day. Such power, such obvious pain.

The heat was becoming unbearable, so we dragged ourselves to the park fountain and its promise of cool water. Off with shoes, the kids are first to dip their feet and splash about. Paul and Gail find refuge under a solitary tree, but we water babies cool ourselves with abandon.

And Jayne, who had just burned the atmosphere with her personal passion, sits quietly on the low edge of the fountain, bare feet in the water, hands scooping and dripping crystal drops, her face completely shaded by a beautiful, wide brimmed straw hat, worn as only Jayne could wear it. With cool contemplation in search of some peace.

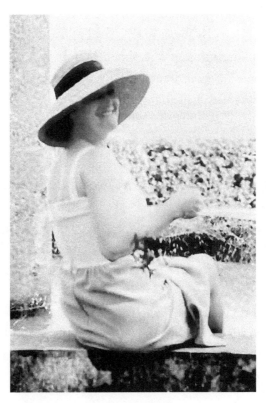

Jayne after her performance at the Burlington Jazz Festival.

*   *   *

Dear Winn' & Doug,

Gail and I attended an evaluation meeting at the home last week. The in-house doctor, head nurse, floor nurse, the home nutritionist, resident psychologist, and mother all sat down with us, and we discussed her situation and addressed her needs. The bottom line is that she seems to be very content.

We had her on a waiting list to be moved downstairs to a nicer area, but when an opening came up, she would not go. She has made a good friend on her floor with whom she attends church regularly. Mother and Ruby have their meals together and get along quite well.

However, her memory is all but gone. She remembers her youth and talks about it more and more, but she doesn't remember Gail's name or know who Jason is. Come to think of it, she never calls me by my name although I know she still knows I'm her son.

She also tells the nurses that she has a daughter who is an actress, but she doesn't know where she lives. She used to ask about Jim all the time but hasn't for several weeks. I don't know where she goes when she wanders into the past.

Love, Paul

*   *   *

It seems a lifetime ago that we left Edinburgh. But it was only seventeen years. I was nine when we took the early morning train to Glasgow and boarded the ship Mardurn. Oh, Mother didn't want to come to Canada. So many tears. Months and months of pleading and planning.

"It's best for us, Jessie," Dad said. "We'll no be alone. My parents and brothers are there, don't forget."

"But my family is here! Please, Jim. Please. Just think how heartbroken Peggy and Mac will be."

Mother was right. Her best friend, whom I called Aunt Peggy, was truly devastated. I remember clearly the last time I saw her. She lifted me onto her lap and hugged me as though she'd never let go.

"You must be brave, Cathy," she said. "Be a good, brave girl for your mummy. She worries about you so." And she cried.

Mother's worry seemed to rub off on me too. I was convinced that the ship would sink, and we'd never see land again. It didn't help that on our second night at sea I was awakened by a great commotion, my parents talking loudly and people shouting in the corridor. The boat was tossing up and down like a cork, and our cabin trunk was floating in water on the floor! I just knew we were all going to drown. Now mother is shouting.

"Jim! Put your leg on! Put your leg on! Hurry up."

A veteran of two wars, Dad had come home safely from both only to lose a leg in a terrible fall while slating a roof.

"Never mind that, Jessie. Help bail!"

Everyone was bailing water. Just where they bailed it to, I didn't know. It was too rough to go up top. Pandemonium throughout the night. It was every man for himself. By morning, the seas had calmed and every steam pipe on board was covered with peoples' clothes drying out.

Dad bought me a treat of Sunmaid raisins from the ship's canteen. Tuppence for the little pack. Mother thought it an extravagance, but Dad said it was my just reward for being so brave.

He's so good to me. Nothing is ever too much to ask. Look how he paid for my Business School classes, my singing classes, and my French lessons, too, even though I'll not be going back to Bathurst to live. I know that now. So does he, I suppose.

But now, after all the false starts, broken engagements, and changes I've been through I finally have a feeling of calm satisfaction.

It's my second year of school and Church work and I'm beginning to think that I've found my long-looked for goal in life. I could
write my diary a year ahead, so sure am I of what I'm going to do!

*　　*　　*

"I've been to Minnie and Peter's farm," my sister admits to me on
the phone. "Oh, Pooh Bray, there's nothing left of it. It's so sad."

"Nothing at all?" I ask.

"Well, the house, such as it is. Just a shell, really. But that's all.
Everything has been ransacked or destroyed. You can hardly find
the laneway, it's so overgrown. I only found it because I knew where
to look."

"I thought they had left everything to some church or charity.
Why didn't somebody do something about it?" I ask.

"I don't know. I know they owed back taxes," Jayne suggests. "I
guess once they were both gone the city took it over and just left it.
Just left it all these years."

"Is the barn still there?"

"No. Nothing, Pooh. There's nothing. It's just a party place. Beer
bottles and litter everywhere. I just stood there and cried."

I can't imagine Minnie and Peter's home like that. Abandoned,
ram shackled. I remember the barn so well. Sunlight streaming
through the spaces in the barn boards, making the particles of hay
dance silently down from the loft. As children we spent a lot of time
there, collecting eggs from random locations in the hay and braving
the leap from the loft to mounds below. No barn.

"Carriage house is gone too." Her voice is touched with melancholy.

"I don't think I remember the carriage house, Jayne. Where
was it?"

"Sure, you do," my sister insists. "It was at the end of the lane,
to the right of the house. You remember. They only had one horse
when we were kids. It died a long time ago, of course. But there was

still a carriage. Just fell apart too, I guess. Or someone stole it." I hear the anger rising in my sister's voice.

"Jaynie, why did you go there?"

"I wanted to see it one more time. I heard that someone bought the land and that they're going to build a subdivision on it."

Now I hear disgust.

"Oh no."

"I did something, Pooh. I took something."

"What? What did you find?"

"Trilliums. I dug up some trilliums and some of Dad's daffodil bulbs and brought them home with me."

Defiance.

"Jaynie, that's lovely."

"That's illegal. You're not supposed to pick trilliums in Ontario, let alone dig them up and take them home. But I didn't care."

"Yeah. Well, you're not supposed to ransack and rob private property either. Or build cookie-cutter houses on beautiful farmland."

I am in solidarity with my sister on this point.

"Do you remember their horsehair couch, Pooh? What an antique."

Her mind is running through a slide show of memories now.

"Is that why it was so itchy? It was horsehair?" I ask. To me the couch had just been a couch.

Thinking back now I realize that the Zavitz farmhouse had been filled with some very rare things that we just took for granted. Things that the family must have brought with them when they crossed the ocean to settle in Ontario. Were they homesteaders? Did Minnie and Peter just inherit the farm when their parents passed away? I had never thought about it. I just knew that we called them Aunt Minnie and Uncle Peter even though they weren't related to us. They had known and employed our Grandpa Percy, or at least their parents had. And they had adored our dad. Once they had wanted to employ our brother Paul on their farm. Mom told me that they needed a boy to help them run the farm and would my parents be willing to adopt Paul out to them? Quit school and work the farm, which he would inherit in the end. What an idea! I guess their mindset was still pretty old-fashioned. Maybe that was when the farm began to fall into disrepair, and in the end, they only had each other and the few ancient necessities of farm life.

My sister and I begin to list the Zavitz family's rare possessions.

"There was a spinning wheel," I say.

"There were three," Jayne remembers.

"Really?"

"Yup. There was small one in the living room . . ."

I interrupt my sister. "That's what I remember."

"But there was another small one and great big one upstairs, too."

"There was? Oh, yeah! I remember the big one now. Was it in the bedroom where we slept?"

"Yup."

"Do you remember the last time we stayed there with Mom?" I ask her.

"I remember the feather bed." Jayne's memory is proving to be much more specific than mine. She had a talent for remembering details. Especially those as pleasant as our times at the farm.

"I remember opening my eyes and seeing nothing at all. It was pitch black. I thought I had gone blind!" I tell her.

Jayne giggles but sympathizes.

"Pretty scary for a little kid, eh? No streetlights, for sure. And you probably couldn't see the stars or the moon for all the trees."

"Yeah, I guess. I never thought about the trees."

And I hadn't until just now.

"They had a stereopticon that they let us look at. Remember, Pooh? All the photo-cards?"

"That was so cool. Remember the pump in the kitchen sink?" I offer.

"Yeah. Minnie thought that was such a modern thing to have." I hear my sister smile. "I guess when Dad lived there you had to use the outdoor pump. That must have been tough in winter," she says.

"No wonder Minnie loved it then. I think the last time we were there with Mom they had built an indoor bathroom too."

"No more double-holed outhouse!" Jayne teases.

"God, I hated that. It was so cold! And scary. I always thought I was going to fall in." That had been a real fear of mine.

"Oh Pooh Bray!"

Now she's laughing. I laugh too.

"And Minnie had a big fur coat that hung on a hook inside the cellar door," I remember.

"It was a beaver coat. Likely Peter's." Jayne says. She's probably right. But how does she know that?

"Well, whatever it was it scared the crap out of me. I opened that cellar door once and I thought it was a bear!"

"Oh no!"

"Honest to God, I swear it moved and growled. I had nightmares about that for ages."

"Oh, poor Pooh Bray. I'm so sorry."

"Well . . . I was pretty young."

"Yup. Long time ago."

We share a quiet moment, each summing up our memories. Then my sister breaks the silence.

"When are you coming home again?"

"Actually, I might take a bit of a mother's holiday this summer if we can swing it."

"Really? Oh, Pooh Bray, that would be so great. Just you?"

"Yeah. Just me."

"Cool. Are you going to stay with Paul and Gail?"

"Maybe for some of the time, but I want to go to Hamilton too. Do you have room for me?"

"Of course! Always. Stay with me. We'll go to Hess Village and the farmers' market. Oh! And there's a new Celtic pub. You'll love it. Wait until you see what I've done in the backyard."

She excited now.

"Why, what have you done?"

"Planted trilliums."

*   *   *

"Mom?"

Paul speaks softly to her as he walks up to the side of her bed.

"Mom, are you awake?"

He told me that she spends a lot of time in bed these days. She rallies for meals and treats, especially milk shakes which she loves. Some people were concerned that milkshakes would cause her to gain weight. But so what? They are full of protein and vitamins, and if she likes them, she should be able to have as many as she likes. That is Paul's opinion. Mine too, come to that.

"She may not know you," he warns. "Don't be upset if she doesn't. Here. Stand here next to your picture."

There are photos over all the walls. A compilation of the family that Paul and Gail created in an effort to keep her memory close. Her four children as well as all her grand and great grandchildren. Larger photos of individual family groupings. And there, beside a few old and yellowed clippings, reviews from long ago performances, was a twenty-year-old promo shot of me; a profile with my hair up and adorned with a cascade of spring blossoms. I haven't looked like that in a long while, but still Paul tells me to stand next to it. Maybe Mom can make the connection.

"Mom?" Paul says. She stirs but does not open her eyes. "Catherine?"

"Catherine?" I ask.

"Yes. Everyone here calls her Catherine because that's the name on all her documents. Sometimes it's all she responds to."

And she does. She opens her eyes and focusses on Paul. She reaches out her hand and he takes it.

"Hello there." She is smiling.

"Hi Mom. Do you know me?"

"Oh, sure, sure. You come to visit all the time."

He smiles. "Look who's here."

"Who?" She doesn't recognize me.

Then Paul points to the photo hanging next to me. "Do you know who this is?"

"Oh, that's an old, old photo."

"But who is it?" he asks again.

"That's me when I was an actress. But that was a long time ago."

"You were an actress?" He has heard this before, I think, but wants me to hear it for myself.

"A long time ago."

The congregation applauds and the Pastor steps forward taking both of her hands in his.

"Amen! Amen! That was wonderful. Thank you, Catherine Smith." She nods her head in a quick bow and steps back to join the rest of the choir. The Pastor continues.

"Let the words of that wonderful song ring out and fill your hearts. 'I would be friend of all—the foe, the friendless; I would be giving, and forget the gift; I would be humble, for I know my weakness; I would look up, and laugh, and love, and lift.'[3]. Friends, that is God's message to us today. He calls on us to be a friend to all. And what better way to share that message than through the song of a young girl whose voice is truly a gift from God."

Cathy sees her mother in the Congregation nodding in agreement. Her dad smiles. He has only come to the service today to

3.   I Would Be True, Hymn, Howard A. Walter, 1906 Samuel R. Harlow (1918)

hear the concert and to hear her sing. He knows that while God may have something to do with her voice, the singing lessons have also been a great gift.

The service is ending now. A final prayer, a benediction and "Go in peace."

"You are really good. You should be on stage."

She's seen him before. His name is Milton, maybe. Or Charlie. But this is the first time they've spoken. He just walked right up to her on the front steps of the church and began the conversation. Mother will not like that. She will not like that at all.

"I don't know anything about acting," Cathy admits. "I just sing in Church."

"But you're really good. You should audition for the Community show in the fall. We're doing HMS Pinafore and they need singers. Besides, you would love it on stage."

"I don't know."

"Cathy!" Her mother has seen her talking to a boy. That is not done.

"I have to go."

"Okay. Maybe I'll see you at the auditions. Just sing that song you did today. You would be great."

"Catherine!"

That is Mother's warning—her full Christian name. Now it's really time to go.

"Yes, I'm coming," she calls to her mother.

Then to Charlie, a softly spoken, "Bye."

"Bye."

Charlie watches her catch up to her parents and waves at her when she turns to look at him once more.

"Catherine?" Paul says gently.

Mom has closed her eyes again and seems to be drifting off to sleep.

"Yes. I'm coming," she mumbles.

She's dreaming. But what of, I wonder? Her lips move as though she is praying. Who knows?

"Are you okay?" Paul asks me.

"Yes. I think so. I mean, I knew she always kind of lived through me, but I didn't know that she thought she *was* me. That's kind of weird. And sad."

"I know. I guess she always wanted to be an actress. So, you're it."

"I guess."

"Let's go get a coffee."

"Okay."

I follow my brother out of the room.

The song was not difficult. It was an easy melody with simple words. And she didn't have to do much more than sing and walk around the stage with her basket. But oh, Charlie was right. She loved it on stage. It won't be her last performance, she's sure. But it will be her favourite because it was her first.

> *For I'm called Little Buttercup*
> *Dear Little Buttercup,*
> *Though I could never tell why,*
> *But still I'm called Buttercup,*
> *Poor little Buttercup,*
> *Sweet Little Buttercup, I!* [4]

"Cathy, that is enough of that silly song. You should be practicing your hymn solo for next week. Here, help me over this field."

They're walking home after Sunday service and taking a short cut across the feral field in front of the church. Cathy takes her

---

4.   The Pirates of Penzance W.S. Gilbert and Arthur Sullivan (1879)

STONE COLD TEA

mother by the arm as she so often does, not necessarily to offer stability or strength. Cathy is no more than a waif next to her mother. No, it was more of a habit. Something for others to see that she was a respectful daughter.

"It was a good show though, wasn't it, Mother?"

"Yes."

"I can't stop thinking about it."

"What's done is done."

"It feels like it was just yesterday, though."

"It is no good living in the past, Cathy. You did the play, but it is well and truly over now."

"Did you think I was good?"

"Don't be prideful, Cathy."

"No. No, sorry."

"The Lord would have you humble in His service."

"Yes, I know. I'm sorry."

Still, she can't stop thinking about how wonderfully fun the whole experience was. And fun was so often in short supply.

"Mother, do you think I might have been good enough to try out for the next show? It's going to be another musical."

"No."

"You think I'm not good enough?"

"No. No more shows or theatre. That is not for you."

"Why not?"

"That way is wildness and shame."

"Do you think so, Mother?"

"I know it to be true, and that should be enough for you."

But somehow wildness and shame did not seem to fit with what Cathy had experienced. After all, their church pianist played the show. And several of the performers were from their church as well. Surely her mother would agree if she just thought about that. But the answer was consistently and firmly,

"No. Certainly not."

205

She should have let it go. She should have just accepted her mother's rule in this, as in all things. But the desire to perform again, to feel that warmth and camaraderie, overruled her common sense and she pleaded.

"I don't understand. Most of the church choir performs in the plays. Why can't I?"

"Because I said so. Because it is not for you." She could hear the impatience creeping into her mother's tone. But still she persisted.

"But why? I just adored singing in the play."

And at that fateful moment everything changed. Perhaps it was a loose stone in the field. Or a clump of dirt or a stick or her mother's own shoe. It did not matter. Her mother's trip was sudden and unexpected. She stumbled forward and just as quickly, regained her balance.

Cathy reached out to take a tighter hold, but her mother shrugged her off, turned toward her sharply and with an open hand furiously slapped Cathy across the face.

"Careless!" her mother seethed. "See how careless you are."

"I'm sorry," Cathy whimpered, holding her hand against her stinging cheek.

"You are careless, foolish, and prideful! You adored singing in the play! You only adore the Lord! You want to go on the stage?! I know what happens to young girls who go on the stage. They get their heads filled with grand ideas. They're beautiful! They're talented! They're better than everyone else! Then they get themselves in trouble and must raise their love child alone!"

"Love child?"

"Yes! Love child! Like you."

What did she just say?

"What do you mean?" But her mother is walking away.

She can't move. She calls out.

"Mother, what do you mean, like me?"

Now her mother stops. She turns, walks directly back to Cathy and stands in front her, her cool attitude almost more cruel than her words.

"You are Aunt Peggy's love child. Peggy, who had a proper Christian upbringing and a respectable steady job wanted to be an actress. To sing and dance and act on stage. So, she acted. Acted like a fool and got herself in trouble. She had no way to raise you, so we did. We took you in just before Jim shipped out and raised you as our own. If that is what you want for your life, then maybe the apple does not fall far from the tree."

The blood drained from Cathy's face, the first slap stinging her cheek and the second burning shame and confusion through her heart. But the greater of these two feelings was shame. She was Aunt Peggy's love child. Mother spoke it with such cold distain it had to be a sin. She was the product of a sinful act—the physical proof of a wrongful deed. And therein lay her shame.

It explained so much. Her strict upbringing. Her endless failed attempts to gain her mother's approval. The lack of connection or any kind of resemblance to her mother's temperament. There had been the constant ache and desire for some form of intimacy. And then the acceptance that she was in some way lacking and undeserving of Mother and of God.

But Peggy, Aunt Peggy was her mother. And Peggy, her mother, loved her. She knew that. Yes. It explained so much. It changed everything.

"Now that is enough. Come. Don't dawdle. Catherine!"

"Yes. I'm coming."

They never spoke of it again.

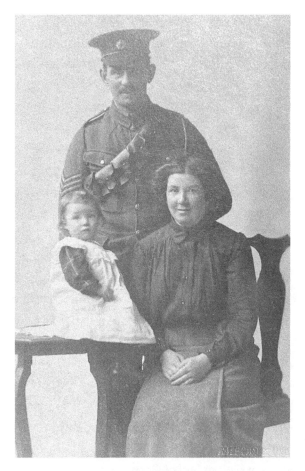

Six-month-old Baby Catherine (1914) with her parents Jessie Stewart Smith and
Sergeant Major James Alton Smith of the 1st Battalion, Royal Scots prior to his
deployment at the outbreak of WWI

*　　*　　*

Jayne was so excited on the phone.

"Did you get my letter yet?" she wanted to know.

"No, not yet."

"Oh, Pooh Bray, wait until you see. I sent you a clipping from the
Hamilton Spectator. It's an entire article about me and my CD!"

"Wow, Jaynie, that's wonderful!"

"Yeah. I got a call last week from Brent Lawson. He heard about the fund raiser they did for me. How Jackie and Jude and everybody performed. So, he called and asked if he could interview me. I said sure! What great promo for the album. I mean CD."

Jayne had called me a few weeks before to tell me about the progress of the recording sessions. Her time in the studio had been enervating. You could hear it in her voice. It was then that she had asked me for a favour.

"Before we press the CD, I wanted to ask you to do something for me."

"Anything." I said. "What do you need?"

"Well, on the CD itself I want to print some kind of dedication. Would you write something for me, Pooh Bray? A poem, maybe? Something that says how I feel about, well, everything."

"Oh, Jaynie. Really?"

"Of course. Who else?"

"What do you want me to write?"

"Whatever you want. Just a few lines from me to my family, my friends, to tell them how I feel about them."

"Wow. I don't know what to say. I'll try."

"Thanks, Pooh."

It took me a few days of thinking and several hours of writing but eventually I sent her four short lines for the CD. And she was happy with them. Now it sounded like it was all systems go for the launch and the extra promotion from the *Hamilton Spectator* would be a boon.

The next day her letter arrived and with it the article.

Its headline read "Jayne Bray's message is her music." And beneath that, "Life hasn't been smooth for this Hamilton jazz singer."

Holy understatement of the decade, I think to myself. No, life sure hasn't been smooth for my sister. But you would never guess that from the photo that occupies a full half of the article. Sitting cross-legged in her office armchair in black slacks, sweater, and thick white socks, my sister beams with confidence and delight. Her soft hair is cropped just below her ears in a classic bob, having recovered from the chemo, and frames her obvious and contagious joy.

It was a human-interest story. The information at the end asked that readers contact the author "if someone inspires you. Someone who has overcome challenges." Well, Jayne's life certainly put her at the forefront as someone who had overcome challenges. In the article, she commented about turning fifty.

"It's been quite a road. That's why I'm so glad to be here, so excited. I've never been so happy to have a birthday in my whole life."

In my heart I can hear her laughter. In my heart I feel a tug of sadness when she says of her cancer,

"I didn't realize I was so important to so many people until this happened to me."

Her CD was entitled *Waltz of Life*. The cover boasted a joyful photo of Jayne dancing with her granddaughter, Karyna. Both in red dresses with no coats, swirling around on a bed of white snow in a dance of pure pleasure, hair flying. One could almost hear their laughter and the music that their happiness sang. On the back of CD case was one of the most beautiful photos of my sister that I had ever seen. Her hair was soft and blond. Her amazing blue eyes deep pools of love and wisdom sorely won. And her perfect smile lit up her entire being with the message that through it all love exists and there is peace in finding your own joy. On the CD itself was the short poem I had written for her.

> To you with whom I've lived this life,
> To those gone in a glance,
> For loving you, my Waltz of Life
> Made sweeter by the dance.

Some of the songs on her CD were old standards. Some were original works by Jayne and her husband and soulmate, Randal.

It was undeniably a musical picture book of my sister's life. Joyful abandon, heartbreak, passion, wit, and sass. The title track and first cut, "Waltz of Life," was an original piece that, as the article states, echoes her feelings.

"Do what you want in life now. Don't wait until the leaves fall and it's over."

The last track and final cut was another original song written with innocence and hope decades before by Jayne and Winnifred Bray.

Down From Above
(The Heavens Open Wide)

Jayne & Winnifred Bray
1961

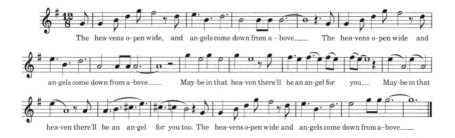

The hea-vens o-pen wide, and an-gels come down from a - bove.____ The hea-vens o-pen wide and an-gels come down from a-bove.____ May-be in that hea-ven there'll be an an-gel for you.___ May-be in that hea-ven there'll be an an-gel for you too. The hea-vens o-pen wide and an-gels come down from a-bove.____

Mom went dangerously vague.
We put her away.
She lives her life now from day to day,
Remembering only moment to moment.
I envy her, she doesn't hurt.
She doesn't know that I've not seen her.
Won't remember when I've been there.
But I remember.

* * *

My grandfather died. This was an experience I shall never forget. Now remember, this is going back to 1919. The night after he died, many people came to the house. We went into his bedroom where he was. The candles were lit and by candlelight he was lifted from his bed and put into his casket. I sat on the window seat with my mother's friend, Aunt Peggy, and held onto her hand with my eyes tightly closed. It was a frightening experience for me. Imagine putting your child through something like that.

* * *

Paul, Gail, and I are sitting in our usual places around the maple wood kitchen table in their home drinking coffee. He looks tired. Worn out.

The funeral is only a few days away and there are still some details to work out. I've brought the photo they asked for. It's a lovely, coloured head shot of Mom from my wedding day. Her hair is beautifully coiffed and she's smiling in semi-profile. Gail will frame it for the service.

The Minister from All Peoples' United will be here tomorrow to talk about the service and to learn a bit about Mom so that she can deliver an accurate and comforting eulogy. She's never met our mom, but Robert Wright, who would have been the obvious choice to preside, is in Northern Alberta and can't make the service. He has sent a message that will be delivered on his behalf.

Paul and Gail have been handling everything for Mom as they have for years. But like a long-distance marathon, the final few miles are the most challenging. Just a few more days now of decisions, organizing, and bottling up emotional turmoil. A few more days and all will be laid to rest with Mom.

"We've chosen the urn. I hope you don't mind," Paul tells me. "It's a lovely marble piece in a pale pink colour. We'll be able to place it in the grave next to Dad at a private family internment."

"That's good, Paul. I'm sure it's lovely. Will it be at the service?"

"Yes. Of course. We'll place her photo next to it."

"That's nice."

I'm glad that people will remember our mom smiling and well dressed. In her independent, younger years she liked to be "well turned out" as she would say.

"About the funeral itself," Paul begins. "What do you think about a viewing? The funeral home needs to know if we'll have an open casket."

"Oh, no. I don't think so."

There is no doubt in my mind about this.

"In fact, I know it's not what she wanted. She told me so many years ago. Why would we need a casket if she's going to be cremated?"

"Oh." Paul seems a bit unsure now. "But people will want to see her, to say goodbye."

"Maybe. But it's not what she wanted. She distinctly told me over many pots of tea. She said, 'When I go, I don't want people standing around looking at my body in a coffin, grieving and crying. It's just a body. I won't be there,' she said. 'I'll be in Paradise with the Lord and happy. I'll be long gone.'"

"She said that?" Paul asks.

"Yes."

"Sounds like her." He doesn't smile.

Now Gail joins the conversation.

"But people need to see her to say goodbye."

"For closure," Paul adds.

"Maybe. But it's not what she wanted."

And I want people to remember her the way she once was. Mom was right. Standing around looking at her body is rather morbid.

"She would want a fond farewell of good memories and lots of music." I add.

"I did pick up a CD the other day. It's bag pipes playing 'Amazing Grace.'"

"That's perfect, Paul."

"Yeah. I've asked that it be played at the end of the service as everyone is leaving."

"Perfect."

There's a pause now. A lull in the conversation as we each sip our coffee and move into our private thoughts for a moment. I break the silence.

"Will the reception be at the funeral home? I've never been to Patterson's. Is their social room on the same floor as the chapel?"

Paul and Gail look at each other, and then he says, "We weren't planning any reception. Just the funeral service and that's it."

"What? Why?"

"Well, we thought we'd just keep it simple."

"But people will want to speak to the family, to each other, and share stories and such."

Now Gail joins the conversation.

"She was ninety. Most of her friends are dead. Who would come?"

Who would come? Who would come! Has Mom's last ten years of fading erased the memory of her from everyone?

"Well, she lived in Welland for sixty-three years. She knew a lot of people," I blurt. "What about her church friends? People from the NDP? The Salvation Army? I'll bet there are still those who were in her cub pack that remember her."

"Cub pack?" Gail asks.

"Yes. Mom was an Akeelah for a scout troop for years. Don't you remember, Paul?"

"Oh yeah." Paul's recognition of this is a soft reply. "I'd forgotten."

"You would be surprised who'd come to Mom's funeral. She wasn't always a ninety-year-old pain in the ass, you know."

I shouldn't have said that. I know what they have put up with these past years while I was far away. I know they need for this to be over. And yes, people need to have closure. But so do I. And my closure involves recognizing the woman our mom once was.

"Well, it's too late to book the funeral home. And it's too expensive there, anyway," Gail concludes.

Paul covers Gail's hand with his.

"Maybe we can find someplace else."

Gail's glance at him says she doesn't agree, and she adds, "Well, we can't have it here."

"No. No, we can't." Then he turns to me. "There might be someplace that's not too expensive. Let me look into it."

"I can help with the expense."

"There's no need. There's still some money in her account that we can use."

"It's too late," Gail says with finality.

But he replies, "We'll see."

I've bought a white photo album and paper that is bordered with roses—pink and white. I've brought several pictures from Mom's old photo album that I have been guarding for years and I spend the evening creating a memory book for people to look at.

Within me a very private war rages. Pictures, vignettes formed out of sequence. Day-old doughnuts, long johns filled with cream from the kind lady at Way's Bakery. The smell of hot, wet cement beneath my chilled and dripping bathing suit. The warm sun on my back. The taste of chlorine on my lips. And the summer sounds from the pool—Ka-thunk! Splash! Squeal!

On the grassy canal bank beside Cross Street pool, she sits with her legs stretched out to the sun, and visits another world, reading *The Good Earth*, a story of China.

The next day Reverend Donna Totten arrives to talk about the service and to learn something about our mom since she's never met her. Paul, Gail, and I answer questions about Mom, her life, her volunteer work.

"I understand your mother was quite a religious person," she says.

I correct her. "Mom would say she would hope to be righteous, not religious."

"A good distinction." Reverend Totten agrees.

"Did she have a favourite Bible story or passage that we might refer to in the service?"

"I don't know," says Paul.

"She loved the story of Ruth," I offer.

"From the Old Testament. Why that story?" Reverend Donna seems surprised.

"She used to quote Ruth saying, 'Whither thou go-est I will go, and where you stay, I will stay. Your people will be my people and your God my God.'"[5]

I can't believe I've remembered that quote.

"So, for her it was about devotion and loyalty?" she asks.

"I guess. Maybe it was about marrying our dad instead of going to the mission fields."

"She wanted to be a missionary?"

"Yes," I answer.

"She did?" Gail asks.

"How did you know that?" Paul seems surprised.

"She told me. We spent a lot of time together before I got married, you know."

"Any other passages or verses you'd like included?"

It sounds like the meeting is wrapping up.

I'm remembering the service for Doug's dad and a wonderful message about clay pots. How the pots may break and crumble away but that we should not grieve the pots. We should celebrate what essence they once held. I can't think of where in the Bible that passage is, and Reverend Donna doesn't seem to recognize it. Oh well. Maybe it's not from the Bible.

"What about hobbies?" she asks.

"Not really," Paul answers.

"She was an avid reader," I say.

---

5.   Ruth 1:16-21, King James Bible

"Yes." Paul agrees. "And she was very active in the community in her earlier years."

"Robert Wright mentions that in the email he sent. He's asked me to read it at the service."

Paul nods. "That's good."

"Is there anything else?"

I feel like I must fill in some blanks here. The total sum of our mother's life sounds a bit thin. What about singing with Charlie Chamberlain from the Don Messer Jubilee? And living in Lethbridge. And riding horses? Helping to haul a threshing machine. What about the CCF meetings she and Dad held when we lived on State Street? She helped Mel Swart get elected. She helped Peter Kormos get elected. She campaigned for the Cancer Society and the Red Shield Appeal. She was an Akeelah. She was a member of Preservation of Agricultural Lands in the Niagara Peninsula. She was a member of the Niagara Peace Movement. She loved theatre. She discovered the Niagara College Theatre Centre, and because of that I went to school there. And she used to show up with sandwiches to feed the students there when we were working on a production. She used to say things like "Take it from where it comes." "The Lord helps those who help themselves." "Bless your stinky little heart." And "I'd rather wear out than rust." Poor Mom. In the end, was she somehow aware that rust was setting in?

As I list her attributes, think them to myself, I wonder how she could have been so misunderstood, so unappreciated by so many for so long. By her family. By me. And I wonder – was this the source of her neediness, her loneliness, the comfort she derived from living in the past? She fought against the passing of her days, clung to the fragments that made up her joy and explained her sorrow and her shame. We were all so busy coping with her while trying to live our own lives, overcome by our own childhood miseries that we neglected to see hers. We failed to recognize the whole truth and embrace the gift of her along with the inconvenience of her. I think all these things to myself. But I do not say them aloud. They become the source of my future shame.

"Well then, I think I have plenty here. Let me say again how sorry I am for your loss. It is never easy to lose a parent, and it sounds like your mother was a unique person. Please let me know if there is anything else I can do for you. You have my number."

Reverend Donna is picking up her valise.

"Thank you," Paul answers for all of us. "Let me show you out."

"Oh, that's not necessary. I'll see you on Tuesday. Goodbye." And she's gone.

"Coffee?" Paul asks me.

"Sure. Thanks."

I am standing by the kitchen sink. Gail is sitting in her spot and Paul is making coffee. As he hands me my mug he says, "We were able to get the Lion's Hall on River Road for after the service."

"Oh good. Thanks. What about food? I can contribute to the cost."

"No, no. Gail's sisters are going to make sandwiches and coffee. It's okay."

"That's a lot of work," I say. "Let me help."

"No," Gail says. "They have it all organized. They have a system. We've done this before."

"Okay." Of course, they have. Gail's family is no stranger to loss. There have been a lot of funerals over the years. Still, I wish I were allowed to help with my own mother's funeral lunch, especially since I insisted on the reception.

Then Paul turns to me and says, "And we've decided to have an open casket."

"No." That's my immediate response. "That's not what she wants."

"It's done. People need a chance to say goodbye." he answers.

What people, I'm wondering. Not me. Paul? Somehow, I don't think so. Certainly not Jayne. Who then? Or is it simply the way it's always done? It doesn't matter. It's a moot point now. The decision has been made regardless of what Mom and I want. I ask Paul if

I can use his computer, and I head upstairs to write a eulogy of my own.

Tuesday arrives. By 1:00 p.m. all of Kay Bray's children and most of their families are here. My in-laws, Nancy and Paul Hartwell ask what they can do to help. I suggest that they transport the flowers from the funeral home to the Lion's Hall after the service. Of course, they will.

At the front of the chapel is the open casket. She looks exactly like the photo I brought from home. Exactly. I suppose that's one of the reasons they needed it.

We begin to greet those coming to pay their respects. A few of Mom's church friends, Mary, Joan, Judy, John, and Susan are some of the first to arrive. Our next-door neighbour from Frazer Street, Ann, signs the book. Robert Stranges who was our neighbour from State Street embraces me and weeps. He is inconsolable. Such a wonderful woman. A wonderful woman, he cries. Peter Kormos comes up the isle to meet me and wraps his arms around me. We stand that way a long while. He can't stay for the service, but he will hold me for as long as time allows. Now Maggie Rumley from River Road arrives. She takes a seat. My high school friend, Greg, whom I haven't seen in decades. He looks the same to me. Friends from All People's United, Ray, Doug, Ron, Terry, the Wights, the Fowlers, and Cathi Bell who went to Riverview School with Jayne and with me. My violin teacher, Bill Murphey. Mitch Jamieson's sister, Marlene, from Burger Street. Now a parade of Jim's buddies from the King Fish and Hunt Club enters en mass. They hug my big brother, offer their condolences to us and leave together.

"That's what we do for each other," Jim explains. "You don't have to tell anyone to come. We just show up to support each other."

And I think that's wonderful.

Now Barb and Bob Nesbitt who live across the street from my mother-in-law are here. Betty Belzner and her daughters have arrived. And so many people that I don't know. More than fifty people have come to say goodbye to Kay Bray, a woman who in some way touched each of them over the ninety years of her life.

The bagpipe music is playing as we continue to greet people. Paul is upset.

"They weren't supposed to play that until we leave."

But I tell him there are a lot of tracks on the CD and we need music. Mom would want music. We'll just have them play "Amazing Grace" at the end.

Now the family is asked to come forward toward the casket and the funeral director closes the partition between us and the other mourners. We stand in a semicircle facing the open casket. No one knows what to do.

Finally, Paul steps forward. "Well, I guess I'll start."

He walks up to the casket, leans over and kisses our mom. Then he goes back to stand with Gail.

Our niece, Karen, is standing next to me. I take her hand. She's trembling.

"Do you want me to go with you?" I ask.

"Yes, please."

We walk together up to the casket, and Karen just stands looking at her grandmother. I lean over and kiss Mom's forehead as Paul had done. It's cold. Stone cold. And hard like marble. This is not my mother. Karen and I go back to our place with the others.

Then Jayne slowly steps up. She stands alone in front of the casket and looks down. Suddenly, from the painful depths of her soul my sister begins to sob uncontrollably. Years of anger, regret, and emotional abandonment boil up through her tiny frame. Why, she seems to be pleading. Why? Her howl is gut-wrenching, and I am helpless to help her. Paul moves quickly to her and holds her to his chest. They cry and tremble together. I hold Karen's hand. No one else knows what to do. Only Paul. I should have gone to her. I should have tried to comfort my sister. Is this what saying goodbye looks like? Is this the closure offered by an open casket?

Now Paul and Jayne move away together and the rest of us calm ourselves. The private mourning is over. When we are seated again in the Chapel the funeral director opens the partition. The casket, now closed, sits centre stage.

The service begins. It's short and sweet. Reverend Donna repeats what we have told her about our mom. She reads Robert Wright's email and then invites Jayne to come up and sing. Poor Jayne. She really didn't want to do this but I pretty much insisted. Mom loved the hymn "The Garden." And Jayne was the singer, after all. There is no accompaniment, but my sister sings it a cappella and flawlessly. I knew she would. Then she sits back down. This day is taking a toll on her as well.

I offer a short eulogy. I talk about how Mom and Dad met. I tell a funny story. I wrap it up neatly and without tears. I am not sure that the mother I have described is the one that my siblings knew. But we've all of us had different relationships with her. I should have said more. I should have reminded everyone who the vital, living, breathing, laughing Kay Bray was. I could have told them how Mom was enamoured of the trees. How she loved to sit beneath them and read. Any breeze that rustled through the leaves comforted her, spoke to her, reassured her that there was a greater nature beyond what she could see. As time stole her sense of time, the trees grew closer to her heart—her mind. I should have told them. But the service is over now.

Bagpipes play "Amazing Grace" as the family stands and goes out into the sunshine. By the time we get into our respective vehicles, Nancy and Paul Hartwell have magically whisked all the floral arrangements off to the Lion's Hall where egg salad sandwiches and hot coffee await us all. There is also tea. Hot and steaming, just as it should be.

* * *

The last time I saw Charlotte Gorbet, we were celebrating her birthday. One hundred and five years old.

"You are my other daughter," she said to me on the phone. "I want you here with the rest of the family."

So we went back east to visit Charlotte again. Over recent years when we visited, she would ask, "Are you coming back next summer?"

"I don't know," I'd tell her.

"Well, I'm not getting any younger," she'd reply in her strong and even voice. Charlotte's voice always sounded to me like confident comfort. Lilting and warm while at the same time entirely practical when logic and practicality were required.

"I'm a hundred and one now, you know. I could go at any time. But if you're coming back, I'll wait for you."

And we'd make the trip. Then in another telephone conversation she'd say, "I'm a hundred and three now, Winnie. I would like to see you one more time."

"We're planning to come."

"Okay, then. I'll wait for you."

I could hear her smile because we both knew that this was our banter.

When Charlotte turned one hundred and five there was no question about whether we would be there. She had recently had a bad fall and had since moved out of her apartment to live with her son, Fred, and daughter-in-law, Charleen, who welcomed us with open hearts and arms.

Charlotte and I spent much of the first day talking, laughing, and reminiscing. It was good to be in her company again, as always. I told her that her family was amazing. That the apple did not fall far from the tree.

"Well," she said. "I have so much nachas. Do you know what that is?"

"No."

"It's a very Jewish word. I don't think there is a single English word for it. Look it up on your phone. Google it."

"Okay." And I pulled my phone from my pocket.

"It's spelled n-a-c-h-a-s," she said.

I found the word quickly enough and I read her the interpretation.

"Nachas is a Yiddish word meaning that you are happy and proud, especially of someone's accomplishments. The traditional wish that Jews offer fellow Jews is 'May you have *nachas* from your children.' *Nachas* is understood to be pride and joy."

"That's right," she agreed. "But it's more than pride. And it usually applies to one's children and grandchildren. I have nachas. But there is no one word in English to describe it."

She smiled. Still teaching me after all these years.

The next day, four generations of Gorbets gathered to be with her and celebrate the world's greatest Mega Bubby! Bubby, because that is the term of endearment for a grandmother. Mega because she was a great grandma, matriarch, and major focus of Love in the Gorbet family.

We laughed and ate and drank. We sang, told stories, and presented all forms of loving honours to her. It was an amazing embrace of Love.

"You, see?" she said. "So much nachas."

When the party ended and all four generations of Gorbets said good night, Charlotte was helped to bed. The next morning, we visited and talked about the joyous day before. She asked me to sing for her again, and I did. We held hands, smiled, and shared a quiet tear for the sorrow of saying goodbye. We kissed.

"I love you, Charlotte."

"I love you too, Honey."

As Doug and I left her room the last thing we heard her say was, "I wonder if these legs will ever dance again."

And she smiled. Content with so much nachas.

You saw me, not with eyes
But with a heart so warm and embracing
It healed and nourished my young soul,
I flourished and grew in your guidance and Love.
Your patience—a tonic to a struggling youth.
And when I could not see my own story
You read my possibilities
And opened the pages of my mind to me,
Gave me hope and dignity.
Because you believed I was worth saving
I found my Worth.
I found my path, my light, my Love.
     Because you saw me with your heart.

*   *   *

Paul sent me an email. I loved hearing from him, and over the years our communication had been steady. He would tell me stories about Welland, family, neighbours, and I would send him accounts of my life in the West. He shared with me his thoughts and feelings about many things, some of which only I was party to, I knew. I did much the same in my letters to him. We were close in mind and spirit. Every year, after his Algonquin Park solo canoe trip, I would receive in the mail a thick envelope stuffed with photos of campsites, wildlife, and peaceful solitude along with his storied accounts of two weeks in the wild. I cherished his thoughtful letters. They were heartfelt and candid, always. But perhaps none more poignant and heart rending than this one.

Hi Winn,
I had a strange dream last night. I feel the need to talk to someone about it but I think it might upset Gail if I tell her – so you're it. Sorry

if this bothers you, but it's okay really. It doesn't bother me at all. Kind of cool actually.

I was at a family picnic at a park somewhere I didn't recognize. Gail was there with Jason, Trudy, and the boys. Jim and Betty with their kids, Mike and Mara, Karen, Shelly, as well as you, Doug, and the kids. Also, Jayne, Randall, and the boys.

I decided to leave and walk to the marina where I planned to spend the night on the boat. It wasn't Sugarloaf Marina, and I don't think it was our current boat. In fact, the entire area was somewhere I've only seen in previous dreams, but I seemed to know the place well. I had to walk along a secondary road to the next concession and I was going to cross to the highway where I planned to walk, or maybe hitchhike to the marina, but there was an old road allowance (just a cart track really) that I took as a shortcut.

As I walked along this trail a huge bear came at me from behind. I turned and fended him off with a kick. He ran around through the brush, circled a few times, and came back at me. I picked up a large stick to hit him with, but it naturally broke into several pieces with the first swing.

The next thing I was aware of was that I was walking down a very narrow hallway towards a small door. When I passed through the door there was another, and then another and another. I was starting to get upset about this when the next door opened out onto a small balcony, something not unlike a castle parapet.

As I stood there, I could see all around the countryside. I could see the picnic area where everyone still was. There were large, open fields, a large body of water with a long, sandy beach and several sailboats offshore.

Suddenly I lifted up and began to 'fly' out over the fields. I moved to where the picnic was and began to hover above everyone. When I realized that they couldn't see me I decided to take on the form of a seagull and began to fly around them.

For some reason, Jayne was able to communicate with me. She asked me where I had been and what happened to me. I told her, "The bear got me."

225

I wanted to let Gail know I was okay, so I changed into an eagle and began to hover over her head, flapping my wings in order to stay in one spot, but this seemed to upset her, so I flew off. Something was trying to hold me back, but I slowly pulled away. Then I woke up. Weird, eh?

Love to all,

Paul

The next day I was talking to my sister on the phone.

"Paul sent me an email about a dream he had."

"The one about the bears?" she asks.

"Yeah. Did he tell you too?"

"Yeah. I sent him a sketch I did of him defeating the bears. He laughed."

"He said that in the dream you were the only one who could see him." A regretful twinge of jealousy creeps into the selfish part of my heart for a moment.

"I know. I know that dream. I've stood on that balcony before," Jayne says.

I remember my sister telling me how when she came out of surgery she asked where her dad was. She seemed convinced that he had been there.

The nurse said, "He's probably in the waiting room."

As Jayne's grogginess cleared, she answered, "That's highly unlikely. He's been dead for forty-five years.'"

"Did you see your dad?" the nurse asked.

"Yes."

"It's okay, Honey. That often happens during surgery."

So now I ask my sister, "What do you mean, you've stood there before?"

"It's okay, Pooh Bray. It will all be okay."

* * *

It's been forty-eight hours since Randal called me.

"If you want to see her before she goes, you'd better come."

It's been thirty-six hours now. We turned her bed so that she can look out the window at the meadow. I've hung the Chinese wind chimes there for her. Just like the ones we used to get at the CNE when we were kids. People have been and gone. Yesterday she rallied and drank a cold beer. But she is near the end now. I've read to her. Jude sang to her. Randal embraces her in both arms. At one point, she wanted to go outside. "I'll take her," I say. But the transfer from bed to wheelchair is too much. We don't make it much past the door. I hold her, bending over the edge of her bed while my high school friend, Daniel, massages the straining muscles in my back.

She's happy I'm here. But she's angry about leaving. I recognize that defiance in my sister. She's not ready. It's too soon for her and she is definitely pissed.

Daniel excuses himself now and leaves me alone with Jayne. When she opens her eyes, I see how tired she is. Not ready, but so done with the struggle.

"It's okay, Jaynie," I say. "It will all be okay."

She squeezes my hand.

I tell her that she is Love and white light. I tell the Universe to accept her beautiful spirit and lift her with joy and peace. Words like comfort, rest, and acceptance form in the close, quiet space between us. Then she sighs, looks up at me and smiles. A small tear escapes from the corner of her eye and it seems her pain is lifted.

Randal is at the door now, so I kiss my sister and step away, leaving her alone with her soulmate.

At the end of the hall is the family room. Sunlight streams through the large windows sending shafts of warm light across the sofas, flowers, and over-stuffed chairs. There is a basket on the hearth of the flag stone fireplace. It's filled with strips of pastel coloured cotton cloth. The little sign in front of the basket invites you to tie one to any tree in memory of a loved one passing. Twice a year they gather all the cloths and burn them in a ceremony of Love, sending the smoke to Heaven, as it were, and releasing the ashes to the wind. I'll do that. Walking out into the meadow beside the hospice, cloth in hand, I walk, passing one tree after another. I don't know which tree I'm looking for or why I think I need to find a specific one. I only know I do. Here. This one. Breathe. There, in the still May air I choose a branch and begin to tie my prayer.

"Open your arms and accept my sister. Let her suffering end. May the Universe gather her and give her flight and sweet release. Go, Jaynie. Fly. Be at peace."

From nowhere a singular, gentle breeze passes through me, fluttering my prayer cloth and teasing my hair in gentle caress. And I know. She's gone. I stand a moment longer holding onto the warmth of her love and I feel a small joy. Her joy at being free.

Back inside, the soft-spoken nurse tells me I had better come. It is very soon now. We stand around my sister's bed—her soulmate, her youngest son, and her one and only sister. Each of us touching her, whispering to her, weeping for our loss as her weary body gives up its last three sighs. The body is gone.

But I know that her spirit has already flown past the pain, danced in my hair, and lifted her in joy to fly away.

* * *

Ever since they told me how short my time may be
Every little sensation has become a delight.
The sky is bigger, brighter, deeper, higher, more touchable
Even when it's Gray, it is a beautiful mystic Gray.
Water colours. The moisture hanging there.
As if it were put there with an artist's brush.
Food
Every little morsel. Each taste.
The bad, a fun experience.

The good. A joy!

Fruit. Sweet, succulent, decadent.

Bread, cheese, an egg, potatoes, a tomato, chocolate

A cup of tea

PASTA............

Water

Oh....... the pleasure of water.

To feel it slip over the lips, caress the tongue. Soothing the throat

Pour it into your hand. Let the fluid crystals drop from
    the fingertips

Feel it on your skin

A breeze on your face

An infant crying

A full belly laugh

Pay attention people!

Delight.

— Jayne Bray

*   *   *

Jim and I were talking on the phone. It had become our habit in recent years to call each other every week or so. In the past we hadn't spent much time together, but now it was only us.

When Mom passed away, I created a photo album of her. Pictures of the woman our father fell in love with. The newspaper clipping describing her on her wedding day. Places we'd lived. Photos of Christmas. Snapshots in time. On this particular day, I had been looking at an old photograph of her four children in winter coats and parkas taken in front of a house where we had lived in Strathroy, Ontario. I don't remember the place. In the photo I'm in a stroller, only one or two years old. But I know that Jayne had a recollection of that time and I tell my big brother about it.

"Jayne always said that house was haunted," I tell him.

"I don't know about haunted," he says. "I know it was hell."

"What do you mean?"

"No heat, no running water. Out in the middle of nowhere. I don't know why we went there. I think Aunt Gertrude or someone she knew, owned it, and we lived there for free. Dad was working at the Sanatorium or something and maybe only came home on weekends. I don't know. I was just a kid. Nine or ten, or something."

"Sanatorium? Where? In London?" I ask.

"No, Byron. I guess that's sort of part of London, now. I think he was working at the Beck Sanatorium, and at the same time he was studying to be a stationary engineer."

"Oh, right. Mom told me about that." I remember. "You know what? I never really thought about it before, but I have one of his textbooks."

"Oh yeah?" Jim sounds intrigued.

"Yeah. It's got his name on the front soft cover and the date 1955. So, I was one in the photo."

"That sounds about right," Jim says. "I guess he was hoping to get work at the hydro station once he finished his course. A good paying job."

"So, how long did we live in Strathroy?"

"I don't know," Jim answers. "A year? Year and a half. All I know is I hated it. Dad was hardly around, and every day Mom sent me to the store in town, six miles away, to buy a loaf of bread or a quart of milk. Every goddamn day."

"You walked?"

"Sure, I walked. Can you imagine that? In those days, a kid walking six miles in the country alone. Boy, you wouldn't get away with that today."

"The photo I have was taken in winter," I tell him.

"Yeah. I walked in winter. Every goddamn day. No boots. Cardboard in the soles of my shoes if you can believe that."

"Oh, Jim."

"Yeah."

"Why didn't she give you a list of things to pick up all at once?" I ask.

"I don't know. Why would she send a kid to do her shopping for her?"

"I don't know."

My brother's childhood memories were so very unlike my own, and I didn't know how to feel about that.

When I look back on our lives as a family, who we once were and what life dealt to each of us, it seems to me that the deck was distributed rather unevenly.

I think that my big brother, Jim, sometimes felt cheated of life's opportunities. He probably would have liked to stay in school if things had been different at home. Like all of us, life handed him his fair share of challenges, some unfairly, some self-imposed. In later years, I began to understand the childhood anger.

Paul planned his own funeral, right down to the music to be played, just to make sure that no one else had to deal with details on top of heart-wrenching loss. He was like that. He felt responsible for everyone else right to the very end.

My big sister, Jayne with a "y," fought for every inch of her self-esteem against every kind of bully. Mental, physical, and emotional. She was served more than her fair share of hurt, harm, and broken heart by loved ones and strangers alike. But the world had not counted on her inner strength and radiant spirit. And when she flew away, she did so with joy and grace.

Herb Bray fell in love with the bolt of lightning that was Cathy Smith. He was English. She was a Scot. She was an Evangelist. He was not. He loved the outdoors, and he had an inherent generosity which made him loved by others. These were his gifts and he shared them until he had nothing more to give. I don't know if he felt cheated.

Cathy Smith, who loved Herb Bray almost as much as she loved her secret friend, Jesus, lived most of her misunderstood life with loneliness in her heart and guilty shame for her decisions. She was wrong to do that. Because despite every blame she either accepted or created, she used all her intellect and many talents to face the challenges life gave her. She did the best that she could. Like all of us, she stumbled from time to time. But there is no shame in that. She loved and was loved.

For the most part, I have lived the life I was dealt without challenging or questioning it, always the baby of the family, naïvely believing we were one, a part of each other, and pushing to prove that to ourselves. But as my loved ones fell away, one by one, I finally faced the reality that my version of our family was entirely my own.

Do we ever really know each other? What are the ties that bind, anyway? And why does it take so long to understand the full tapestry of our lives?

I tug on a thread of shame here, darn a hole that is regret there, and dab at the stains that mar our memories. And in the end, it is not a good cup of tea that solves everything.

It is forgiveness. Especially of ourselves.

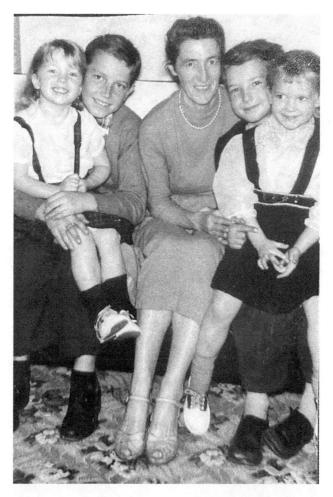

Kay Bray with her children (1961) left to right, Winnifred, Jim, Mom, Paul, Jayne.

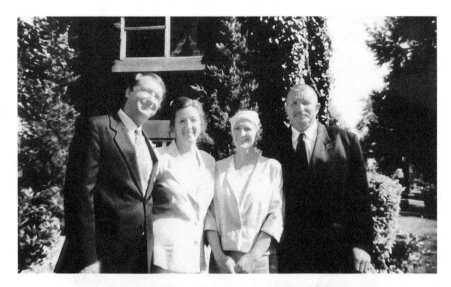

The Bray siblings. Paul, Winn, Jayne, Jim (1999)

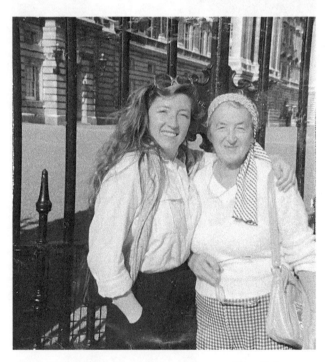

With Mom in London, England where, in Russell Square,
where we enjoyed the best cup of tea we ever had. (1984)

THANK YOU TO . . .

Douglas J. Rathbun, my husband, best friend, and steadfast rock, whose support and belief in me is, and has always been, unwavering. The love of my life.

Our incomparable adult children, James Rathbun, and Heather and Orin Rathbun Bishop, whose many talents provided photography, music transposing, recording, computer and marketing support, patience, encouragement, and permission to share.

Vern Thiessen, who guided me through the process of finishing this book, offering invaluable insight, suggestions, encouragement, and support.

Lynn and Ron duFort, whose incredible friendship and selfless support is unique in the world. Lynn, who first suggested that I finish the manuscript and who, with Ron, read and reread draft after draft, keeping me on course.

Lana Skauge, master storyteller, author, and playwright whose positive spirit, moral support and encouragement was, and is always, just a phone call away.

Kathleen Speakman, Heidi and Denis LeClaire, Ann Barrett and Don Pitman, and Dorothy Bishop, who read the first draft and offered very helpful feedback.

Michel Paquet, who proofed the French language dialogue.

Susie Moloney, whose workshop was encouraging and instrumental.

Bryce Allen, who provided valuable research information.

Kevin McKendrick and Glenda Sterling, who supported the project.

Charlotte Gorbet, my friend and teacher, who never doubted my ability and encouraged me to follow my heart.

ACKNOWLEDGEMENTS

Alberta Foundation for the Arts
Writers' Guild of Alberta
Edmonton Public Library Writers in Residence Programme
Calgary Public Library
Welland Historical Museum
Corporal William Franklin, Canadian Armed Forces
Jill Smith, Forces War Records, Edinburgh
Canadian Museum of Immigration, Nova Scotia
Canadian Historical Railway Association, Niagara
John MacFarlane, Directorate of History and Heritage, Canadian
    Armed Forces
Niagara Military Heritage Centre

ABOUT THE AUTHOR

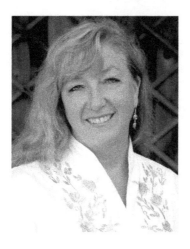

Winn Bray Rathbun has been a professional playwright for more than three decades, with fifteen produced plays and musicals to her credit. Her work has largely focused on historical drama, theatre for young audiences, and telling unique Canadian stories. She was the recipient of an Excellence in the Arts Award (Hamilton Wentworth Creative Arts), and her work has been recognized and supported by, among others, the Ontario Arts Council, the Alberta Foundation for the Arts, Heritage Park and BMO Financial Group, Quest Theatre, Lunchbox Theatre, Mount Royal University, Alberta Playwrights' Network, duFort Enterprises, Carousel Players, Theatre South NSW (Australia), the Citadel New Play Development Program, and the private sector.

Winn Bray Rathbun currently lives in Calgary, Alberta. *Stone Cold Tea* is her first published book.

Printed in the USA
CPSIA information can be obtained
at www.ICGtesting.com
JSHW022332120424
61038JS00007B/23